T0262851

HEALTHY, WEALTHY, OR WISE?

HEALTHY, WEALTHY, OR WISE?

Issues in American Health Care Policy

CHARLES T. STEWART, JR.

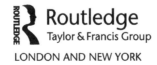

Routledge
Taylor & Francis Group

LONDON AND NEW YORK

First published 1995 by M.E. Sharpe

Published 2015 by Routledge
2 Park Square, Milton Park, Abingdon, Oxon OX14 4RN
711 Third Avenue, New York, NY 10017, USA

Routledge is an imprint of the Taylor & Francis Group, an informa business

Library of Congress Cataloging-in-Publication Data

Stewart, Charles T., 1922–
Healthy, wealthy, or wise? : issues in American health care policy /
Charles T. Stewart, Jr.
p.   cm.
Includes bibliographical references and index.
ISBN 1-56324-504-3 (hbk.).
ISBN 1-56324-505-1 (pbk.)
1. Medical policy—United States. 2. Medical economics—United States.
3. Insurance, Health—United States. 4. Medical care, Cost of—United States.
I. Title.
RA395.A3S82   1995
362.1′0973—dc20   95-6892
CIP

ISBN 13: 9781563245053 (pbk)
ISBN 13: 9781563245046 (hbk)

Contents

Preface

For many years I have been concerned about the overemphasis on medical treatment in the maintenance of good health.[1] Medical care was, and remains, inefficient. But what precipitated work on this book was a foreboding that the sustained upward creep in the share of gross national product (GNP) going to the health care industry would erode the living standards of my children's generation. I fear for their future, when in the second decade of the twenty-first century the post–World War II baby-boom generation achieves retirement age. At that time, living standards could experience a sharp drop.

I am concerned about health costs, not over the next few years, but in the next thirty years. With continued growth in technology, in the population over sixty-five years of age, and in medical care costs, this industry, which absorbed 5.3 percent of GNP in 1960 and now takes 14 percent, is projected to absorb nearly one-third of GNP by the year 2030.[2] We could be spending almost as much on other health care issues: environmental health and household and workplace safety. These large increases in share of GNP devoted to health care imply a decreasing share of private income available for other goods and services; they also mean that most government expenditures will be needed for health care, social security, and interest payments on the debt, with little left for anything else. Resources available for private investment and research other than medical research will be reduced, slowing economic growth. Living standards will have to fall if radical change is not implemented fairly soon.

This book examines the varied causes of the rapid increase in the cost of health care over the past three decades and considers the transformation of our health care delivery system that must occur early in the twenty-first century if private standards of living are not to decline and all other government social and economic programs are not to be starved. Proposals under discussion today would not reduce health care costs. They might slow down the future rate of increase, but that is not enough; that simply puts off for a few years the consequences outlined above. The share of GNP devoted to health care is excessive now, and it must be cut.

What follows is not a proposal about specific policies but an analysis of what must be done if health goals are to be attained without sacrificing everything else: why and what, not how. The obstacles in the way of a wise use of health care resources are not the difficulties in deciding what we want, although our wants often conflict with one another. Nor is our main problem ignorance of how to get from where we are to where we want to go. The principal obstacle is the opposition of powerful groups who stand to lose, or fear they may lose, from the radical reorganization of the health care industry needed to safeguard living standards and achieve a more productive use of valuable resources.

I have talked to many people about the issues raised in this book. Some of their ideas, information, and experiences are reflected in it. I should mention my wife, Nancy Thayer, my daughters, Eileen and Jocelyn, and my sister Anna Louisa McCartney, who made substantive contributions as well as providing moral support. Richard Scheffler will be surprised to know that conversations some years ago made a contribution. Mary Ann Baily and Thomas Moore are a continuing source of information and insight. They will not agree with everything I say, and I retain the same right toward them. To repeat a confession I heard many years ago from Walter Buckingham of Georgia Tech, I agree with myself at least 90 percent of the time. But all the facts are never in. On some minor issues my mind could be changed in the future. But not on the major findings and conclusions.

Notes

1. Charles T. Stewart, Jr., "Allocation of Resources to Health," *Journal of Human Resources* 6 (Winter 1971): 103–22.
2. Sally Burner, Daniel Waldo, and David McKusick, "National Health Care Expenditure Projections through 2030," *Health Care Financing Review* 14, no. 1 (Fall 1992): 1–29.

1

Determinants of Health

¡Salud! Skoal! A votre santé! To your health! Drinking alcohol is no longer recommended, but the universality of the salutation bears witness to our ever-present concern about our health.[1] There must be something we can do about our state of health, besides drinking toasts in its service; otherwise our concern would be misplaced. In fact, our health is the outcome of four basic determinants:

1. Our genetic endowment, over which we exercise no choice at all, although our parents may have had it in mind
2. The environment in which we live, over which individuals usually have no control, although they may choose to change environments, but over which individuals organized for collective action can exert substantial influence
3. Our lifestyle, over which we can exercise substantial choice, within the constraints of the second determinant
4. Health care, including the treatment of departures from good health and preventive measures other than changes in lifestyle and environment

The Determinants of Health

Genetic Endowment

Individuals cannot influence their genetic endowment. Nevertheless, it may change over time, through choice of mates or through differential mortality and fertility rates. Natural selection has played a major role in resistance to illness. The isolated populations of the Americas proved highly susceptible to measles, tuberculosis, and various infectious diseases that were relatively mild in populations exposed to them for many generations. The survivors were those with greater natural resistance, which they tended to transmit to their offspring. A similar effect was the outcome of the Black Death in Europe in the fourteenth century.

Our knowledge of the genetic basis of disease is in its infancy. As we learn more, it may become possible to calculate rough probabilities of the incidence of various cancers, diabetes, some forms of mental illness, and the propensity to various other ailments on the basis of individual genetic endowment, as well as the chances of passing them on to our offspring. Decisions on whether or not to have children, and with whom, are ultimately moral, not medical, decisions. To the extent that such decisions are influenced by genetic considerations and treatment possibilities, health is only one among many desiderata.

All of us have some genes not conducive to the best of health or to long life. We are just beginning to learn how to correct for some genetic deficiencies through transplant techniques. In some distant future we may exercise some control over our genetic endowments by direct medical intervention. With the progress of science, genetic propensities toward disease need matter less and less. Lifestyle and environment, both largely within our individual or collective control, and both beyond the jurisdiction of the health care industry as we currently know it, will grow in relative importance. We know less about the implications of lifestyle and environment than we do about the infectious diseases that were the main threat to health and life in the past. Perhaps they matter less.

Environment

Which genetic traits are undesirable from a health standpoint, which desirable, depends much on the environment and our state of knowledge. The sickle-cell mutation is Janus-faced; in a malaria-ridden environment, it confers an advantage; elsewhere, a risk of high blood pressure and strokes. Intolerance of milk and dairy products, common among Asiatic people, is of no concern in environments in which milk and dairy products are rarely consumed but contributes to infant mortality in other environments. Once we become aware of the problem, it is no longer a problem—there are substitutes for milk.

Awareness of the influence of a pure water supply goes back a long time. So does the first successful experiment with vaccination. One changes the environment, the other protects individuals from environmental hazards. Traditional prevention refers to clean water, sewage disposal, safe food, vaccination. Early in this century, these were the main contributors to improved health and longevity. More recently, prevention has come to include product safety, workplace health and safety, and a reduction of environmental pollution. Exhaust emissions from motor vehicles and factory and power-plant smokestacks have received the most publicity, but many other harmful emissions and toxic wastes have also come under regulation. Industrial progress has created new environmental threats. Environments may be changed: the Environmental Protection Agency (EPA) and the Occupational Safety and Health Administration (OSHA) are designed to do this on a large scale, but individuals can do some things for themselves; for example, adding humidifiers, filters, and fireproofing to their homes.

Lifestyle

Health can be maintained by preventing illness; health can be restored by curing it. Many of the cancers, strokes, and heart attacks experienced today could have been prevented; "prevented" may not be the right word, but postponed certainly, for we all die of something someday. In addition to public efforts at prevention via environmental change, individual efforts via behavior modification have also increased. New industries of aerobics and many other forms of exercise, as well as health clubs, have blossomed. Dieting, whether by individuals in isolation or in clubs, even under the supervision of specialists in nutrition, has become fashionable. So has the consumption of vitamins, minerals, and other dietary supplements. The recent decline in average cholesterol levels and blood pressure may be one outcome. The sharp drop in smoking is another example of a behavioral change designed to minimize chances of illness.

Medical Treatment

Most diseases are self-limiting; others, such as arthritis, are chronic, essentially incurable, at least for now. Medical treatment can make a difference in only a small proportion of these chronic cases, and this only recently.[2] In the past, medical treatment on a net basis did more harm than good; this situation may not have been reversed until this century—some would say until the arrival of sulfa drugs and antibiotics. Substantial earlier progress was attributable to vaccination, a safe water supply, better sewage disposal: public health measures, rather than medical procedures.

Diabetics can live fairly normal lives with appropriate diets and/or insulin. Hemophiliacs can rely on blood-clotting agents and transfusions. Progress is being made on some cancers and on cardiovascular disease. Many metabolic deficiencies may be readily counteracted by medication. And we are just beginning to learn how to correct for some genetic deficiencies through transplant techniques. But differences in mortality and health levels between the United States and other industrial countries, and differences within the United States, are primarily related to genes, environment, and behavior, not to the quantity or quality of medical care.[3]

Research

Research can change any of the basic health determinants. Right now, there is little we can do about genetic endowment beyond making decisions about reproduction. But we are learning more about the genetic basis of illness and disability, enabling us to improve our chances of avoiding them. Eventually we expect to correct some of the genetic causes of disease. The prospect that we will be able to "cure" bad genetic traits exists, but we should be wary of the American belief that technological outcomes are certain if we only spend enough money on them. The ill-fated war on cancer should dampen our faith somewhat. Research contributes in a major way to better treatment, as well as to behavioral change and environmental modification to improve health and reduce chances of illness. It is responsible for most of the large increase in life expectancy since World War II. How much money is spent on research, and how it is allocated between these determinants of health, in the long run determines what gains are made in quality of life and life expectancy.

With the growth in knowledge, we face wider choices: constraints on lifestyles, resort to available treatment, environmental modification, eventually even genetic change. But health is only one among many considerations. The role that physicians and the health care industry had in the days when infectious and contagious diseases were the dominant concern and antibiotics were developed to treat them will never be the same again.

The agenda of health is undergoing revolutionary change, as a result of past achievements and new knowledge. As we gradually eliminate transmissible disease, through public health measures preventing epidemics, through vaccination, through education; as we learn to identify the harmful features of our environment and proceed to cope with them, whether by prevention (clean air and water legislation) or by improving our methods of diagnosis and treatment (early detection and treatment of a variety of precancerous and early cancerous conditions, antiallergen drugs, treatment of burn and accident victims) or by protective measures (safety belts, smoke detectors), more and more of the burden of disease becomes attributable to our genetic endowments and our personal lifestyles: diet, exercise, smoking, stress. It may appear anomalous that at the very time when the role of medical treatment should be declining on the health agenda, as a result of previous achievements and increased social and individual preventive efforts, there has been a rapid increase in expenditures on medical care and quantity of medical services rendered. Why have the amount and cost of treatment increased so rapidly?

The concept of disease and health is a relative one. As our general state of health improves, so do our standards, our levels of aspiration. Humans are problem solvers; if there are no old problems outstanding, they must invent new ones. Obesity, alcoholism and other forms of addiction, various mental states or behavior patterns that in other societies are associated with poets, creative artists, and holy men become objects of medical concern. Whether they are or are not medical problems is not the issue; the point is that conditions and behavior formerly not regarded as of any concern to the medical practitioner, or perhaps to society, have been added to the medical agenda.

This expanded scope for medicine reflects in part the secularization of life, the decline in prestige or acceptance of other professions and role figures: religious leaders, spiritual and moral counselors, the *pater familias*. We seek a doctor's prescription, chemical salvation, instead of earlier forms of solace or help. In part, the expanded scope for medicine is the legitimate result of breakthroughs in the therapeutic arts: diseases or conditions formerly untreatable, and untreated, such as epilepsy or diabetes, now are modifiable or manageable.

A major aim of this book is to understand why expenditures on medical care have been increasing so much more rapidly in America than in other advanced nations, and why per capita health expenditures in the United States are considerably higher than anywhere else, even though by measures of longevity and infant mortality Americans do not fare as well as most industrial nations. A second aim is to examine the efficiency of health care delivery and consider whether health care resources are properly allocated between and within prevention, treatment, information, and research. If we understand the underlying causes of cost increases, and the productivity of several health care approaches, then and only then can we know what needs to be done to reverse these cost increases, which is our final aim.

Of all the professional services, three have names for their customers specific to the service rendered: the lawyer has clients or listeners; the recipient of educational services is a student, for study is what he or she does. The customer for medical services is a patient, from the Latin word for suffering, because that is what the patient does—in body or mind or pocketbook or all three. But suffering is not intrinsic to the art of healing, as study is to learning. So there need be little further use of the pejorative term "patient." Those in the hands of would-be healers will be called "customers," which is what they are.

Notes

1. The Chinese, I am told, are an exception; they drink first to your wealth, not to your health. It seems that no people drink to wisdom first.

2. Victor Fuchs, *Who Shall Live?* (New York: Basic Books, 1975), 64.

3. Ibid., 6.

2

Why Are Costs
Out of Control?

The Price of Health Care

Basically, this book is not about cost and price but about values. Nevertheless, the choices between values that confront us when discussing health care would not have to be made were it not for the high and rising cost of that care. In 1960 the nation devoted 5.3 percent of its gross national product (GNP) to health care. Three decades later, in 1990, it spent 12.2 percent of a GNP that had more than doubled in the meantime. By 1993, the share rose to 14 percent. Our real expenditures on medical care have quadrupled. Even allowing for population growth, per capita real expenditures for health care have nearly tripled.

No one would claim that we are receiving four times, or even three times, as much health care as we did in 1960. There have been some gains: substantial increases in longevity for those over age sixty-five, lower infant mortality, and a more equitable distribution of medical care. Since 1965, most of the poor have gained better access to medical care, as indicated (inadequately) by number of visits to doctors' offices. Could these gains not have been achieved without more than doubling the share of income going to medical care?

First, let us look at the big picture: the large increases in health care spending, the inflation in prices. (In Chapter 3 we look briefly at future projections under the current system and the implications for economic growth and living standards.) Second, we examine briefly in this chapter the particular causes of mushrooming medical costs and their interrelations.

The growing share of GNP devoted to medical care is presented in Figure 2.1. These estimates are on the low side; they are not comprehensive. They do not include much of the expenditures on public health. They exclude some research and development costs, which will contribute in the future to improved public health. Where does one draw the line? Expendi-

Figure 2.1. **Expenditures on health as a percentage of GNP.** From U.S. Bureau of the Census, *Statistical Abstract of the United States* (Washington, D.C.: Government Printing Office, various years); and *Historical Statistics of the United States from Colonial Times to 1980* (Washington, D.C.: Government Printing Office, 1975).

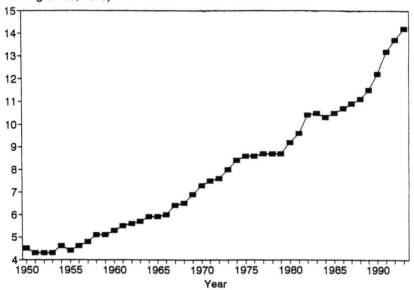

tures on public health whose main if not sole objective is prevention and improved health should be included. Should we then include expenditures on environmental quality? Air-pollution control? Workplace-pollution control? What about workplace safety and product safety expenditures? The list is long. The distinction may be between prevention of disease and prevention of accidents. There is no hard-and-fast line; both require medical care. The point is that it is not just health care expenditures in a narrow sense that have been increasing; practically every category involving environmental hazards at home or workplace or in products, whether "disease" or "environment" or "accident," has been increasing. There are some common causes underlying these increases. They deserve some of the credit for reduced mortality and must bear part of the negative consequences for economic growth and living standards (Figure 2.2).

Share of Employment

The medical care industry employed 8,871,000 workers in 1993 (plus 262,000 in health insurance); it was our second largest industry, behind retail trade (see Table 2.1). In 1950 health care workers numbered 1,239,000. The

Figure 2.2. **Trends in medical and consumer prices (1982–84 = 100).** See Figure 2.1 for sources.

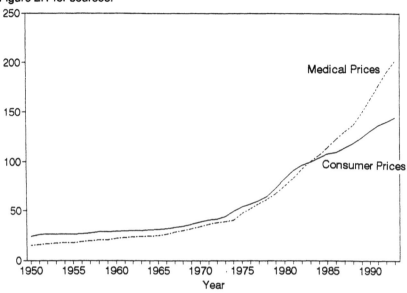

Table 2.1

Employment Trends in Medical Care

	Medical Care Workers	Percentage of Total Employment
1950	1,239,000	2.1
1960	2,054,000	3.0
1970	3,130,000	3.9
1980	5,278,000	5.2
1990	7,814,000	6.7
1993	8,871,000	7.3

Source: U.S. Bureau of the Census, *Statistical Abstract of the United States* (Washington, D.C.: Government Printing Office, various years).

health care industry share of total employment rose from 2.1 percent in 1950 and 3.0 percent in 1960 to 7.3 percent in 1993.

If one were to include employment in firms supplying a wide variety of products to the health care industry, as well as private-sector and government employees working with health insurance, the number would be substantially larger. Although the health care industry share of employment has risen, it has not risen nearly as much as its share of personal income. Pay for health workers has risen much faster than in the economy as a whole, one aspect of cost increases. The industry constitutes a powerful lobby against effective control of medical costs, since such control would entail the loss of many hundreds of thousands of jobs, possibly a million or two, and reductions in pay for some and slowdowns in pay increases for others.

International Comparisons

What about the output resulting from this great increase in health care spending and employment? To be truthful, there is no measure of overall output or productivity. More on this later. But some industrial countries spend less than half as much as we do as a share of GNP, most of them less than half as much per capita (Table 2.2). Most industrial countries fare better in terms of life expectancy, even though they have universal health coverage and their elderly population comprises a larger share of their total population than ours does. For example, the population sixty-five years of age and older in the United States was 12.6 percent in 1991, whereas it was 12.8 percent for Japan, 15 percent for France and Germany, 15.1 percent for Italy, 15.4 percent for the United Kingdom, and 17.9 percent for Sweden. Even countries with a reputedly high percentage of hypochondriacs— France and especially Japan—do much better than the United States. It does not appear that we are getting much return for spending so much more than other nations. If there is a relationship between health care spending and life expectancy among advanced countries, no one has been able to detect it.

The health care costs of other industrial nations are not only much lower than those of the United States but are increasing much more slowly. In fact, some countries—Denmark, Ireland, Sweden—experienced a real decline in medical costs as a share of GNP between 1980 and 1991; others had minimal increases (less than 0.5 percent of GNP)—Austria, Germany, Japan, the Netherlands. In more recent years, the United Kingdom and France also experienced a decline in their share of GNP devoted to health care.

American medicine is said to be the best in the world. That may be true. It has pioneered in many diagnostic procedures and therapies; it provides many high-tech, costly services rarely available elsewhere for wealthy people all over the world, financed in part by our taxes and health care premiums. We hear anecdotes about cases of indifference, mismanagement, incompetence—you name it—from Germany, the United Kingdom, and other advanced countries with health care systems our medical lobbies do not like. One can find similar anecdotes here. A German or an Englishman might even cite the enormous number of malpractice suits as evidence that

Table 2.2

Health Expenditures, Selected Countries

	Share of GDP (1991)	Per Capita (1991)	Life Expectancy (1993)
United States	13.4	$2,867	75.8
Australia	8.4	1,407	77.4
Austria	8.4	1,448	76.4
Belgium	7.9	1,377	76.7
Canada	10.0	1,915	78.0
Denmark	6.5	1,151	75.5
Finland	8.9	1,426	75.7
France	9.1	1,650	78.0
Germany	8.5	1,659	76.1
Greece	5.2	404	77.5
Ireland	7.3	845	72.2 (1991)
Italy	8.3	1,408	77.4
Japan	6.8	1,307	79.2
Netherlands	8.3	1,360	77.6
Norway	7.6	1,305	74.1 (1991)
Portugal	6.8	624	74.9
Spain	6.7	848	77.5
Sweden	8.6	1,443	78.1
Switzerland	7.9	1,713	78.0
United Kingdom	6.6	1,043	76.5

Sources: U.S. Bureau of the Census, *Statistical Abstract of the United States* (Washington, D.C.: Government Printing Office, 1993), tables 1383 and 1376. 1991 Statistics for Ireland and Norway are from *World Health Statistics Annual.*

our system does not perform well at all. The point is that in a large country one can find examples of anything. But examples do not reach a conclusion. What is the performance of different health care systems, as measured by output, not by anecdotes? The answer is that Germany, Canada, and practically all advanced countries do better on health care than the United States, as indicated by the output measures of longevity and infant mortality—and at much lower cost. One might reply that medical care is by no means the only determinant of infant mortality or adult longevity. Given the superior performance of the health care systems of other industrial nations, perhaps some, or much, of the money we spend on health care might be better allocated to other determinants of health and longevity. This is not to imply that the United States should cut its health care spending in half; other nations are not without their problems. But it does imply that something is badly wrong with a system if it is so out of line with every other advanced nation. Perhaps we can reduce health care costs to levels comparable to those of other countries with no sacrifice in terms of performance. Clearly, we are wasting much of our money.

Price or Quantity of Services?

Suppose that since 1960, when only 5.3 percent of a much smaller GNP was spent on health care, there had been no price or pay increases in the health care industry in excess of general inflation. In 1993 we would be spending on health care not 14 percent but 10 percent of GNP. Thus, roughly 42 percent of the increase in share of GNP spent is due to price increases and 58 percent to increases in quantity of medical services delivered (assuming that price indices over such a long time period accurately measure price changes). Why such a large price increase? Why such a large increase in quantity? Population growth was 42 percent—much less than GNP at 75 percent; it cannot account for the increasing share of the GNP spent on health care although it does account for most of the 58 percent increase in quantity. The increase in quantity of services alone should have resulted in a *decreasing share* of GNP going to health care.[1] The increasing proportion of people over age sixty-five—from 8.15 to 12.5 percent—by itself cannot account for much of the increase. Thus most of the cost increase was the result of higher prices, not greater quantity per capita. Why did the share of GNP devoted to health care grow more than 150 percent since 1960, even though real GNP per capita increased 75 percent during this period?

Edgar Peden estimates that between 1965 and 1990, prices for medical care rose 1.5 percent a year above the general inflation rate; quantities of medical services rose 2 percent a year above the GNP growth rate.[2] Victor Fuchs estimates these changes between 1947 and 1987: health care prices increased 1.6 percent a year more rapidly than other prices, whereas quantity grew 0.9 percent more rapidly than other quantities.[3]

Is the price increase justified? How much of the additional quantity of health care, beyond that explained by growth in population and its changing age distribution, is reasonable, representing tests and treatments not previously available, some for conditions not previously treatable? How much represents an increase in overtesting, overtreatment? It is not easy to answer these questions. The increased proportion of the population in older age groups requires increased delivery of medical care, but how much of an increase? One estimate is that a 0.3 percent annual increase, or one-third of Fuchs's increase in quantity of health care between 1946 and 1986, can be attributed to changed age distribution of the population.[4] Much of the increased spending in fact has been on customers over sixty-five years of age, but was the increase appropriate or excessive?[5]

Causes of the Huge Cost Increases

Why have health care costs increased so rapidly, more than doubling their share of GNP in thirty years and showing no sign of slowing their growth?

First, there are the demographic causes of increased demand: a rapid rise in the number of people over sixty-five, seventy-five, and eighty-five years of age, groups that are much more intensive users of medical care than younger people, and in the proportion of the population in these age groups. This increase in medical care has been happening already, but most of the impact is still ahead, particularly when the post–World War II baby-boom generation reaches sixty-five (Table 2.3). The increase in numbers, and in share of the population, reflects in part high birthrates in the past and their decline in recent decades. But it also reflects improvements in public health and medical care that have sharply reduced infant mortality and increased life expectancy in older age groups. Of those born around 1920, only half survived to age sixty-five; this figure is expected to rise to over two-thirds for those born around 1950, and four-fifths for those born around 1990.

There are three visits to a doctor and/or hospitalizations for a thirty-year-old to every one for a twenty-year-old; there are five for a forty-year-old, eleven for a fifty-year-old, and twenty-six for a sixty-year-old.[6] A smaller proportion of the population, those under age ten, also have a higher proportion of health care needs than the population as a whole. On a net basis, the change in age composition has increased the need for health care. Nothing can be done about this.

Another aspect of demographic change has increased the demand for health care and especially for hospital care. The decline in birthrates means that aging people have fewer children to look after them than they did in the past. The availability of Medicare and private insurance weakens the motivation of children who might help if no alternative was available. The proportion of families with single parents has risen dramatically. If the single parent works, who stays with sick children? If the single parent is ill, who looks after that person? The proportion of two-parent families in which both parents work has also increased, again hampering home care for children or for a parent who is ill. The change in living arrangements from an extended family living under one roof or in close proximity to the nuclear family with at most two generations under a single roof, often far removed from close relatives, combined with greatly increased labor-force participation by women and high geographic mobility, has made it inconvenient and

Table 2.3

Trends in the Elderly Population

	Number 65 and over (000's omitted)	Percentage of Population
1960	16,675	9.2
1970	20,085	9.8
1980	25,550	11.2
1990	31,061	12.4
2000	34,886	12.8
2010	39,704	13.4
2020	53,627	16.6
2030	69,838	20.2

Sources: U.S. Treasury Department, *Statistical Abstract of the United States* (Washington, D.C.: Government Printing Office, 1994); *Historical Statistics of the United States* (Washington, D.C.: Government Printing Office, various years); Dennis Ahlburg, "The Census Bureau's New Projections of the U.S. Population," *Population and Development Review* 19, no. 1 (March 1993): 169.

often impossible to care for the sick at home. The increasing number of older people living alone has shifted much health care from home to hospital. The urbanization of what was largely a rural society improves access to medical and especially hospital care. Monetization of health care, formerly part of the household and family subsistence economy, is no different from buying vegetables in a supermarket instead of growing them yourself. Some of this shift occurred because the market alternative was subsidized by the government or covered by insurance, whereas the household options were not.

Second, the passage of Medicare and Medicaid legislation in 1965 extended medical services to millions who had been inadequately served or not served at all and allowed suppliers of health services to charge low-income patients who had received free services. The eligible population receives more health care than it would have received in the absence of such legislation, since the cost of Medicaid services to the customer approaches zero and that of Medicare is 20 percent of the Medicare-approved price. There is no change in need, but there is an increase in use. No one argues for the elimination of these programs unless a substitute can be found to replace them. But they help explain the large increase in health care spending in the late 1960s and early 1970s, although not the continuing rise since that time (Table 2.4).

Third, the proportion of the population covered by private health insurance increased from one-tenth in 1940 to one-half by 1950, 72 percent by

Table 2.4

Growth of Medicare and Medicaid

	Expenditures (billions)		Percentage of Health Expenditures	
	Medicare	Medicaid	Medicare	Medicaid
1967	4.5	2.9		
1970	7.6	5.2	11.1	7.9
1980	37.5	23.3	16.6	11.3
1990	112.2	75.2	17.3	11.7
1992	137.7	129.3	17.3	16.3
1993	151.1	112.8	19.3	14.4
2000	327.6	359.8	19.3	21.2
2010	862.9	744.8	23.3	20.1
2020	1,950.0	1,442.4	25.4	18.8
2030	4,133.9	2,856.2	26.3	18.2

Source: Health Care Financing Review, Fall 1992, 26–27; Fall 1994, 285.
Note: Figures for 2000, 2010, 2020, and 2030 are estimated.

1960, and about 86 percent today. The share of third-party payments in personal health care expenditures rose from 34.5 percent in 1950 to 60.5 percent in 1970 and 76.7 percent in 1990 (these figures include payments by Medicare and Medicaid as well as private insurance companies). This again has no effect on need, but it does have a large delayed effect on demand. Whatever happens to the price charged to the insurance company, to the customer it is zero or close to a free service. No one is arguing for the elimination of health insurance. But as we see in Chapter 4, the prevalence of third-party payments influences all other causes of increased costs.

Population aging, Medicare and Medicaid, and private health insurance—these three factors account for much of the increase in demand for health care in recent decades.

Fourth, the slowdown in economic growth after 1973 and the long recession of the late 1980s and early 1990s contributed to the rise of medical costs as a share of GNP (but not necessarily to increase in demand). But causation runs both ways. The rapid increase in health care spending and in insurance premiums may have slowed growth and partly accounted for the failure of real wages to rise. This effect is considered in Chapter 3.

The traditional American expectation that economic growth will solve all problems is not going to be realized. We have maintained growth recently by greatly expanding the proportion of the adult population (women) in the labor force, with serious side effects for the well-being of the family, and have come close to the maximum size of labor force attainable given our adult population and given the pressure to postpone entering the labor force by prolonging schooling. The share of income saved and invested has fallen, and static or declining real incomes do not result in more saving and investing. We already have 7 percent less of the GNP available for investing than Japan, and the shortfall will soon be 10 percent or higher. (Much of the increase in health care expenditures is now consumption, not investment.) Even during past periods of rapid growth, health care expenditures rose more rapidly than GNP; with slow growth in GNP, the share going to health care grows even more rapidly.

Fifth, there has been a growing tendency to oversupply medical services of all kinds: tests, treatments, drugs. The United States may not be number one in life expectancy, but it is number one on a large number of tests and surgical procedures performed per capita. A major explanation is the large increase in the ratio of physicians to population, from 14 per 10,000 in 1960 to 23.4 in 1990. Why more doctors should result in more tests and more operations per capita is discussed in Chapter 5. There are explanations, but no justifications other than so-called defensive medicine, which is a response to the huge increase in malpractice suits, malpractice awards, and therefore premiums for malpractice insurance. Since the insured customer is insensitive to cost and ignorant about benefits, it is easy for supply to create its own demand.

Although new technology required some increase in the number of M.D.s, as well as some increase in the ratio of specialists to general practitioners, the growth is increasingly generating a surplus. New medical school graduates, about 16,000 a year, are far in excess of replacement and growth needs, and this figure does not consider foreign medical school graduates (many of them Americans) who are entering practice and now constitute about 20 percent of all practicing physicians. New graduates have exceeded replacement needs for more than twenty years, so the average age of M.D.s has fallen, and the surplus will take a long time to shrink. Too many surgeons result in too much surgery; too many doctors increase the use and drive up the price of medical services.

The reasons given so far help account for the large increase in the amount of health care delivered, apart from prices, although they may also contribute to rising prices. The additional reasons given below help explain the steep rise in prices.

Sixth, increases in medical incomes have far exceeded those for other professions (Table 2.5). Increases for other health care industry workers have also outpaced the rest of the workforce, although not to the same extent. The

Table 2.5

Trends in Earnings, Physicians and Others
(Employment Cost Index, 1981 = 100)

	Physicians' Earnings (000's omitted)	Index	Index		
			Health Care Workers	Professional and Technical Workers	All Civilian Workers
1965	$28.9	33.6			37.3
1970	41.5	48.1			47.0
1980	83.7	97.1			92.2
1981	86.2	100.0	100.0	100.0	100.0
1982	93.3	107.9		109.4	107.5
1983	104.1	120.8		115.9	114.5
1984	108.4	125.7		123.8	120.8
1985	112.2	130.2	122.7	128.7	126.4
1986	119.5	138.6	127.5	134.0	131.5
1987	132.3	143.5	133.4	138.6	135.9
1988	144.7	167.8	140.3	145.6	142.1
1989	155.8	180.7	148.9	152.6	148.9
1990	164.3	190.6	159.5	162.2	156.9
1991	170.6	197.9	168.6	170.5	164.1
1992	177.4	205.8	176.3	177.3	170.0

Sources: Calculated from U.S. Bureau of Labor Statistics, *Employment Cost Indices and Levels*, nos. 2389 (1991), 2434 (1993) (Washington, D.C.: Government Printing Office, 1991 and 1993); American Medical Association, *Socioeconomic Characteristics of Medical Practice 1994* (Chicago: AMA, 1994).

increases can be described as another example of supply-side economics. The ability of providers to increase demand for their services has permitted growing surpluses without falling incomes; on the contrary, in many instances, the greater the surplus the higher the price, compensating for some reduction in average workload.

The National Center for Education Statistics provides data on college and university faculty salaries for academic years 1962–63 and 1987–88. In the earlier year, health services faculty earned an average of $7,789, whereas physical sciences faculty averaged $9,213 and biological sciences $8,689. In 1987–88, positions were reversed: health services faculty earned much more than natural sciences: $50,900 versus $37,000 in private institutions, $53,500 versus $41,000 in public institutions.[7] The National Institutes of Health pays more for M.D. researchers than for Ph.D.s in the same positions, although the latter are trained in research, and the former may not have been.

Table 2.6

Pay of Tenured NIH Scientists

Occupation	M.D.	Ph.D.
Investigator	$83,249	$67,131
Section chief	89,653	76,819
Lab chief	95,185	89,827

Source: Traci Watson, "Task Force: Level the Playing Field," Science 260 (May 14, 1993): 888–89.

Between 1980 and 1990, while real hourly earnings in all industries declined 6 percent, and in services increased 5.2 percent, in health services real hourly earnings rose 14.5 percent, and in hospitals, 22.6 percent.[8] Between 1990 and 1993, hourly earnings in health services continued rising much faster than elsewhere in the economy.

Defenders of physicians' earnings point out that they constitute less than 20 percent of medical costs. That is really irrelevant because the principal impact of M.D.s on medical costs is not their fees but their decisions on volume of services: tests, procedures, hospitalization, most of whose costs are not doctor fees but are means of increasing physicians' incomes. It is estimated that physicians account for 70 to 80 percent of medical costs. Each additional M.D. raises medical costs by over $800,000 in addition to his or her own pay. Defenders also argue that medical earnings are not too high; they represent only a reasonable return on investment in very expensive medical education, perhaps including in these costs the relatively low earnings during internship and residency. Since the largest cost element in medical schools is the salaries of the faculty, this argument amounts to saying that physicians must have high earnings because physicians have high earnings.

Seventh, diagnostic tests and treatments have been developed that did not exist in the past: CT scanners, MRIs, coronary surgery, pharmaceuticals for depression, kidney dialysis, and organ transplants, to name only a few. Medical conditions that went untreated now fall within the province of the health care industry. Some new technologies increase the quantity of medical services; others increase prices.

Technologies that improve on existing treatments tend to reduce costs, whereas those that treat conditions previously untreatable, that extend the scope of medical care, tend to increase costs. (But the assumption that untreatable conditions do not absorb health care resources is not always true. We have no treatment for influenza but nevertheless examine and hospitalize; there is much expensive care, even if there is no cure. Pneumonia also was costly before antibiotics offered a cure.) Smallpox, polio, pneumonia, tuberculosis were eliminated or reduced as threats to life and health by vaccines and antibiotics, which greatly reduced the cost of these illnesses. Prospects of comparable magic bullets for cancer and cardiovascular disease (and for AIDS) are remote; what new technologies have done is moderate illness or prolong life at increasing cost.

New technology has become less cost effective. Too much of it is very skilled labor or capital intensive: MRIs and heart surgery, for example. Too much of it benefits a limited number of individuals, by contrast with the measures that practically eliminated many dangerous epidemic diseases of the past or greatly reduced their cost, such as penicillin and vaccines. The illnesses that constitute a growing share of medical needs, such as cancer and cardiovascular disease, have not yielded to effective preventives or cures but are treated with expensive new "halfway" technologies. A cause of concern is new technology that permits the protraction of dying but not the prolongation of life among the very old, and among the not so old who could not survive without life-support systems and intensive medical care, and new procedures that neither prevent nor cure but are marginal improvements over existing procedures—and are much more costly.

Eighth, the high price of drugs is often mentioned as a culprit. I think not. First, the cost of drugs as a share of total medical costs has decreased dramatically over time, from 13.6 percent in 1960 to about 7 percent today. Second, the average price of drugs, until the mid-1980s, increased much less than the average price of all medical services. Third, the use of drugs often avoids the need for more expensive procedures, such as cardiovascular surgery. Drugs are poorly covered by health insurance policies, one reason why they are so much in the public mind. If they were to become adequately covered, one could expect higher prices and greater use of drugs, hence increased total amount spent on drugs and more research and development by pharmaceutical companies, more new and new me-too drugs.

Prices for drugs in the United States are higher, often much higher, than prices for the same drugs abroad. There is excessive competitive spending on research, resulting in too many new products scarcely different from one another, and excessive spending on advertising in competition for the same therapeutic markets. The cost of developing new drugs increased greatly after changes in Food and Drug Administration (FDA) requirements for approval of new drugs in 1962, but any continuing increase in cost is attributable to scientific and technological difficulties and to the threat of litigation, rather than regulation.

Ninth, there is excess demand for new technologies that have resulted in costly excess capacity that in turn has led to overuse. There is the technological imperative, operating in the past, the present, and the future, which on a net basis drives up the costs of medical care. This extra cost arises from complex motives both on the part of physicians and on the part of their customers. The demand for novelty is deeply embedded in the ideology of progress that has prevailed in this country since its inception. It can be reduced, although it is not an easy thing to accomplish. There is too much faith in the physician as miracle worker and not enough awareness of the physician's limited role in treating many conditions. The customer, over the years, has raised levels of expectation about health and well-being; aches and other departures from perfect health that were once tolerated now lead to demands for cure.

Tenth, larger administrative costs are often cited. Many people seem to believe that 1,500 health insurance companies and the health care deliverers dealing with them have no bureaucracy; only governments do. In fact, the health insurance industry is the most expensive health care bureaucracy in the world by a wide margin. One recent study defining administrative costs very broadly concludes that administrative costs are 24.8 percent of total hospital costs.[9] The Department of Health and Human Services suggests that it should be 15 to 16 percent. Constantly changing regulations and the existence of so many health care insurers add to confusion and cost. But one purpose of many administrative costs is to place some restraint on the quantity and the price of medical services. It has not worked very well, and the existence of competing insurers and competing providers is the main reason why restraints have been ineffective.

What will happen to administrative costs depends very much on the organization of health care delivery and compensation in the future. The shift of health care from a cottage industry to a hospital-based factory system has greatly increased administrative costs both for operating the system and for cost reimbursement. Much inefficiency and waste could and should be reduced, particularly on the cost-reimbursement side.

Eleventh, litigiousness, to which the insurance coverage of health care deliverers contributed, has in turn contributed to the growth in cost of health care insurance coverage. In 1986, a peak year, one of every three physicians was sued. The oversupply of lawyers is no doubt a factor. Popular misconceptions about what medical care is and what it can be expected to do are others. The amount of premiums paid is a partial indicator of the cost of litigiousness. The physician's time is another. Excessive testing and excessive treatment, however, are more difficult to pinpoint and are much more important. They are in part a change in behavior responding to the risk of litigation, a change that should moderate the rise in health care deliverer insurance costs by reducing the risks of successful litigation. But they may simply shift upward the standards of care, with little effect on the probability of being sued. But the change in behavior is in part a response to the opportunities for profit generated by third-party payments. Some defensive medicine, and some malpractice suits, are nothing but greed masquerading under the pretense of self-insurance or self-defense or fair compensation. Malpractice premiums are sometimes dismissed because they account for only 2 percent of total medical costs. More relevant is the fact that they are nearly 10 percent of physicians' incomes, and much more than that for the specialties at high risk. The average premium paid by M.D.s in 1990 was $14,500; for surgeons, $22,800, and for ob/gyns, $34,300, amounts that more than doubled since 1983. The average income of M.D.s in 1990 was $164,500. If physicians were not able to pay high malpractice insurance premiums, they would be much less tempting targets for hungry lawyers and discontented customers, juries would not be recommending preposterously large awards, and it would be more difficult to make a case for the practice of "defensive" medicine.

Another reason for the increase in malpractice suits is the proliferation of new technologies and the failure of some physicians to use them or to use them properly. The need for almost continuous learning by and retraining of M.D.s is much greater than it was in the past. A literate population and a premature proliferation of articles on new technologies in professional journals and the popular press have greatly increased public awareness of new and possibly effective approaches to old diseases.

Twelfth, there has been a change in the structure of the medical care industry. At the time of the last revolutionary reform in medical education, the outcome of the Flexner Report in 1910, which responded to the growing scientific base of medicine, the practice of medicine was conducted primarily by individual M.D.s in their offices and in the homes of their patients. One-fourth of the population was still engaged in farming, and most of the rest lived in rural areas and small towns. Now the preponderance of medical care delivery is conducted in institutional settings: hospitals, clinics, group practices. Even the individual solo practitioner is likely to work in conjunction with other M.D.s and supporting paramedical personnel. The administrative costs of a solo practice are becoming prohibitive. A largely rural population has become predominantly urban, and the accompanying vast improvements in transportation and communication have made possible the use of centralized health care delivery facilities. The proliferation of tests and treatments involving expensive and bulky equipment, a wide range of supplies, and the trained personnel to conduct tests and operate equipment have made the individual practitioner's little black bag a subject for humor. Institutionalization has become a necessity. Health care delivery has become a large and complex industry that M.D.s are poorly prepared to manage either by training or by inclination.

A simple way of summarizing the change in structure of the health care delivery industry is to consider the change in its workforce. Early in the century, most of the workers in the industry consisted of M.D.s. Today, for every M.D. there are thirteen other workers. The growth in health care delivery employment is in part a shift from home-based health care, in which individuals providing nursing and aid to nurses were members of the family, not counted as employed in health care. But much of the growth in employment is net growth, not a shift from households. Changes in the structure of medical care have also contributed: the decline in number of primary-care M.D.s relative to the population and the surplus in many specialties have shifted treatment to specialists that might have been handled by general practitioners, and to hospitals rather than to outpatient units, both shifts raising costs considerably.

There are further reasons for the growth of hospital-based health care. Hospitalization is a way of providing reimbursement for "house calls," which otherwise might not be covered by insurance. It is a device for consolidating house calls so as to economize physician time and travel. Hospitals play a custodial role, including provision of hotel and restaurant services, for patients too sick to look after themselves who do not have household help; they are a means of reimbursement for convalescent homes and nursing homes that are covered by insurance only if a patient is sent to them from a hospital. The overbuilding of hospitals has resulted in cost increases and overuse.

Finally, the health care industry is labor intensive; services are usually delivered on a one-to-one basis. William Baumol tells us that such service industries advance more slowly in productivity than industries with a much higher ratio of capital to labor, where substitution of capital for labor is easily done.[10] There is something to be said for this argument. Nevertheless, Baumol's recent statement on changes in the real price of health care for eighteen industrial nations identifies three—the United Kingdom, France, and Finland—where real prices fell over the 1960–90 period, and a fourth, Denmark, where prices did not change. Sweden had only a 0.1 percent rate of increase, and Japan, Italy, and Spain had 0.4 percent rates of increase. Furthermore, the divergence between health care prices and other prices in the United States should be observable as far back as one cares to go, but in fact seems to have developed in the 1960s. A fundamental problem is that we have no overall measure of the productivity of health care in this or any country. Surely there are more medical workers per patient in hospitals than before, but what of it? We have mentioned demographic, technological, and institutional changes that make it impossible to compare these ratios over any significant number of years. How many coronary bypasses were there in 1960? The difference between health care and education is the rapid change in what economists call the production function in the former: from aspirins to antibiotics, from bed rest and crutches to cardiac and orthopedic surgery, as well as major changes in product: cures where none existed previously. Education has experienced little change in production function since Aristotle; its product changes, but nowhere near as fast as in health care. Another way of looking at it is the change in the labor mix: before World War II, there was one health care employee per M.D.; now the ratio is thirteen. In education, most employees are still teachers.

Prime Causes: Technology and Insurance

In listing the various components of the cost increase of health care, one should consider that some are not independent of each other, but interact. Because of this linkage, allocating shares of cost increase to particular causes is an oversimplification. For example, the increased cost of health care for the elderly is largely a function of new and improved technology for dealing with the typical problems of the aged. On the other hand, an increased share of research and development devoted to the problems of the elderly is partially explained by their increasing numbers, which in turn are partially explained by improvements in public health measures, vaccination, and antibiotics long ago, as well as by more recent technology that has prolonged lives. Thus an increased share of research and development devoted to the elderly is one result of successful previous research and development. New technology has contributed to the greater specialization and higher incomes of M.D.s, and hence greater numbers of M.D.s. Availability of insurance coverage increases incomes of M.D.s, which increases the numbers of M.D.s and encourages an oversupply of services.

The main culprit of increased costs of medical care is the growth of third-party payments, which affects all the other culprits, even age distribution. We are not going to reduce the extent of third-party payments; on the contrary, most plans propose to extend them to all those not at present covered. The really important interaction is that between increased private insurance coverage plus Medicare and Medicaid on the one hand, and increased excess demand, increased fees and prices, higher salaries and earnings, oversupply of medical services, overutilization of facilities and equipment, and increased spending on research on the other. The relation is predominantly unidirectional.

The second culprit is technological progress, which continues independently, but which has been heavily subsidized by insurance coverage, which widens the markets for its products. In combination, technology and insurance greatly increase the supply of medical services and the demand for them, almost regardless of price. It is to these four components of cost increases and to their interrelations that we devote the following chapters.

Future Trends

What about the future of prices, fees, the excess supply of medical services, and the other factors driving health care costs? We should distinguish between causes that will continue to increase costs and those whose elimination would not reduce their rate of increase, only result in a one-time decline. Of all the causes of increased share of health costs in GNP, which are likely to persist? Excess demand and excess supply of services are largely the result of the growth in insurance coverage, which will not grow much more; they cannot continue increasing forever. Neither can the excess supply of M.D.s or the prices for their services. It is not conceivable that administrative costs will continue increasing indefinitely.

The cost of malpractice litigation (including the practice of "defensive" medicine), which is passed on to customers, should decline. Ceilings on the size of awards and on the share going to lawyers, already in place in some states, are likely to become national, reducing the incentive to bring suit, the costs to insurance companies and the health care customer.

Aging of the population will continue into the mid-twenty-first century. What it will mean for medical costs depends largely on future technological progress and the extent to which it improves health versus prolongs life, as well as future practices on the high cost of dying for a few.

Universal Coverage

Some 37 million people, or 15 percent of the population, are not covered by health insurance, are under age sixty-five, and are not poor enough to be eligible for Medicaid. The percentage covered has actually fallen slightly in recent years. These people are primarily the self-employed and workers in small firms, and their dependents, as well as some of the unemployed and a few dependents of workers who are themselves covered but have not obtained coverage for members of their families. It is reasonable to assume that most of those lacking coverage will receive it in some form in the years ahead. The impact on total costs of covering an additional 15 percent or so of the population should not be exaggerated. Most already receive medical care, too often expensive emergency-room care. Some pay for their care, mainly those who are young, healthy, and deterred by the high premiums of individual health insurance policies. The costs of those who do not pay are largely borne by the rest of us in higher prices and insurance premiums and higher taxes. One estimate puts the increase in office visits and hospital admissions at 4 percent and the increase in total costs at 2 percent; another puts the increase in costs at 4 percent.[11] But this is more a once-and-for-all increase than a continuing cause of rising costs.

Many who are covered have coverage that is too limited to handle protracted illness or major medical costs. There may be insurance coverage for catastrophic illness, but its impact will be small compared to the impact of Medicare and Medicaid. More complete coverage, and coverage of more people, both increase medical expenditures. When one adds up the consequences of coverage for catastrophic illness, coverage for an additional 15 percent of the population, and somewhat broader coverage for large numbers, the total increase in medical expenditures from these sources alone could be substantial, but finite, not continuing indefinitely.

Most of those currently uncovered do not have the advantage of employer-based group health policies and would have to pay individual rates, which are often twice as high. Simply making health insurance available to all at community rates might substantially reduce the number uncovered and reduce total expenditures for health insurance for those who pay individual rates, some of whom might opt for higher-benefit policies than they now hold.

New Technology

Trying to predict new technology and its impact on health care costs is mere speculation. Early in this century, large gains were made in reducing infant and child mortality (more as a result of public health measures than of medical treatment). In midcentury, the main gains were from antibiotic treatment of bacterial infections, reducing health care costs. Recently, progress has been made in reducing deaths from stroke and heart attacks, diabetes, and kidney failure, most of them affecting older individuals with greater than average health care needs. Most of the treatments themselves are expensive. Improved technology for existing ailments may well come at increasing costs and diminishing returns. One area where breakthroughs could result in large savings is the development of antiviral drugs. Whether or not, or when, this will come about, no one knows. The bacterial antibiotic revolution seems to have largely run its course, with the development of resistant strains of bacteria and allergic reactions to many antibiotics, both accelerated by the overuse of antibiotics. Another prospect for reducing medical costs is the development of a vaccine protecting against malaria, which may be close to attainment, although nearly all the beneficiaries would be in Third World countries; in this country malaria epidemics were eliminated by public health measures many decades ago. There is much talk and research on vaccines for AIDS, but these are measures to delay the onset of the final stage by boosting the immune system. An effective treatment or a preventive vaccine does not seem to be imminent.

Expanded scope for treatment will grow: in the case of geriatrics, we should expect diminishing returns but continued progress at high cost. The new area of genetic therapy is hard to predict, but it does offer the prospect of reducing health care costs by eliminating some genetic ailments such as Parkinson's disease that result in chronic illness and improving preventive and early detection measures by identifying individuals genetically most prone to serious ailments.

Any effort to understand the future of the industry must ask whether technological progress will contribute more to widening the scope or to improving the effectiveness of medical care.

Prevention

Although the scope for treatment will expand, and the ability to treat will improve, the need to treat should decline. The trends we have seen in lifestyle, stressing healthy diets and regular exercise, should continue, reducing rates of strokes and heart attacks. The decline in smoking and excessive drinking of alcoholic beverages should continue. We are less certain about future use and abuse of cocaine, heroin, and other psychoactive drugs. As our understanding of the effects of industrial chemicals at work, at home, and in the general environment improves, we will move more effectively to control their use or human exposure to them. The incidence of some cancers should decline. And there is the prospect that genetic therapy will prevent some illnesses and perhaps prevent the inheritance of the propensity for some illnesses.

Thus the main continuing causes of rising medical expenditures are new technologies, the excess demand for them, and the tendency of suppliers to overuse newly developed tests, equipment, procedures. Some of the increase in share of GNP devoted to health care can be justified, and we would not wish to reverse a combination of technological and social progress. But we would be better off if future increases were from a lower base, a base rid of excessive compensation, excessive prices, overtreatment as a result of malpractice fears on the one hand and technological imperatives on the other, excess demand on the part of customers who are risk averse and well insured against the costs of treatment, and finally, bloated administrative costs. There are other concerns: health care resources are badly allocated and their productivity is low and could be greatly increased.

Notes

1. Victor Fuchs, *The Health Economy* (Cambridge: Harvard University Press, 1986), 281.
2. Edgar Peden and Mei Lin Lee, "Output and Inflation Components of Medical Care and Other Spending Changes," *Health Care Financing Review* 134, no. 2 (Winter 1991): 75–81.
3. Victor Fuchs, "The Health Care Sector's Share of the Gross National Product," *Science* 247 (February 2, 1990): 534–38.
4. Division of National Cost Estimates, Office of the Actuary, Health Costs Financing Administration, "National Health Expenditures, 1986–2000," *Health Care Financing Review* 8 (Summer 1987): 1–36.
5. Estimates of the contribution of prices and quantities to increase in cost of medical care are based on the difference between the Commerce Department medical price indices and the index of consumer prices. These ratios are approximate. There are problems in estimating the medical price index over long time periods. The biggest is the result of new technology. New procedures are introduced, diagnostic as well as therapeutic, and new pharmaceuticals enter the market. Some employed in the early period disappear from the market or drop in significance. In some instances the prices for new drugs and equipment drop as their market expands, production costs decline, patents expire, substitutes are developed. The case mix also changes, with changing age distribution, in technology, access to insurance, but also as a result of improved prevention. For instance, there has been a drop in heart attacks and strokes. This complicates estimates of long-term trends in quantity of medical services.
6. Stanley Wohl, *The Medical Industrial Complex* (New York: Harmony Books, 1984), 45.
7. National Center for Education Statistics, *Digest of Education Statistics* (Washington, D.C.: Government Printing Office, 1964 and 1991), table 176.
8. Gregory Pope and Terri Menke, "Hospital Labor Markets in the 1980s," *Health Care Financing Review* 9, no. 4 (Fall 1993): 127–37; see esp. 131.
9. Steffie Woolhandler, David Himmelstein, and James Lewontin, "Administrative Costs in U.S. Hospitals," *New England Journal of Medicine* 329 (August 5, 1993): 400–403. See also David Himmelstein and Steffie Woolhandler, "Cost without Benefit: Administrative Waste in U.S. Health Care," *New England Journal of Medicine* 314 (February 13, 1986): 441–45.
10. William Baumol, "Social Wants and Dismal Science: The Curious Case of the Climbing Costs of Health and Teaching," C.V. Starr Center for Applied Economics RR #93–20, New York University Department of Economics, May 1993.
11. Stephen Long and Susan Marquis, "The Uninsured 'Access Gap' and the Cost of Universal Coverage," *Health Affairs* 13 (Spring 1994): 211–20. See also Brenda Spillman, "The Impact of Being Uninsured on Utilization of Basic Health Care Services," *Inquiry* 29 (Winter 1992): 457–66.

3

Must Living Standards Decline?

Projections of Health Care Costs

The reader may wonder why there is so little reference in this book to the detailed proposals for health care reform that were a major subject of public debate in 1993 and 1994. The reason is that there is little or no prospect that what needs to be done will be done in this century. In fact, the Clinton administration proposals anticipated an increase, not a decrease, in health care costs, and offered only the very-long-term prospect of slowing down the rate of increase in costs. What needed to be done was considered politically impossible or prohibitively costly. The big losers would be most (not all) of the medical profession, hospitals, and insurance companies, which are wealthy and well organized; whereas the prospective winners were too many and too small and too ignorant to be organized into comparably effective lobbies.

Any honest program to lower costs and slow their rate of increase will cost many jobs, certainly over a million and perhaps more. Most of the insurance companies' 268,000 employees would go, as would a sizable proportion of the administrative employment in hospitals and other providers of health services. There would be losses among health care personnel as well, perhaps substantial losses. A new health care program would also lower many incomes. Is it any wonder that there was all-out resistance?

The share of GNP devoted to health care is certain to rise in the years if not decades ahead, which means the money will not be going to other desired purposes. The Health Care Financing Administration, which is required to make projections, has had to raise its estimates repeatedly. In 1987 the projection for the year 2000 was 15 percent; in 1991, it was 16.4 percent; in 1992 expenditures were projected to reach 18.1 percent of GNP in 2000, and 32 percent in 2030.[ ] Projections have been subject to an upward creep, as reality has repeatedly outrun expectations. Victor Fuchs said in 1990: "Many expect the United States share to reach 15 or 20 percent within a few decades."[2] William Baumol estimates that we will be spending over 35 percent of GNP on health in the year 2040.[3] A projection is not a prediction, just a warning of what may happen if something is not done, and done sooner rather than later.

If one looks at the distribution of medical costs by income group, the impact on living standards is already substantial. The top 5 percent of the income distribution pays, via premiums, taxes, and out of pocket costs, only 10.2 percent of its income on health care; but the bottom two deciles pay respectively 26.9 and 20.5 percent.[4] These figures exclude nursing home care and nonprescription drugs.

Looking at government rather than household expenditures, increased spending on health, mainly Medicare and Medicaid, and on social security are already crowding out other programs. One estimate is that social security and Medicare, accounting for 13.7 percent of taxable payroll in 1992, will rise to 25.2 percent by 2030.[5] The health insurance (Medicare) component of payroll taxes is currently 2.9 percent, no longer enough to cover costs, which are projected to rise to 3.74 percent of payroll in 2000 and 8.62 percent in 2030. Federal government expenditures for health care were less than 5 percent of the total federal expenditures in 1965, 15.4 percent in 1990, and are expected to rise to 28.8 percent in 2000; state and local government expenditures were 8 percent in 1965, rose to 12.5 percent in 1990, and are expected to rise to 18.8 percent in 2000.[6] And the proportion will keep on rising into the next century. This has implications for the public standard of service. If one adds to the rapidly rising share of public revenues going to health care the also rapidly rising share going to social security and state retirement programs (enlarged by the impact of health care on life expectancy), plus the growing interest payments on a growing national debt, there is no way that other public services can grow; in fact, there is no way to prevent their decline.

Estimates by the Office of Management and Budget of lifetime tax rates for successive generations with current health care programs find that generations yet unborn will face tax rates of 82 percent, versus 29 percent for those lucky enough to have been born in 1920.[7] Obviously this will not happen; the people will not stand for such rates; benefits and costs will be cut, and better sooner than later. But the political power of the groups that gain from the present situation, or stand to lose from necessary reforms, is such that necessary radical changes are likely to be too late, and too little. There will be social disruption and intergenerational war.

An Aging Population

Two consequences of advances in medical treatment are that a larger proportion of the population is reaching age sixty-five and that there is a longer life expectancy for those who do. The proportion of the population sixty-five years of age and older, which was 9.8 percent in 1970, rose to 11.3 percent in 1980 and 12.5 percent in 1990 and is projected to reach 20.2 percent in 2030 and then creep up to 20.6 percent in the next twenty years (this is the median projection, which on the basis of past experience may prove too low). This age group is afflicted with chronic diseases, often treated at great expense, with incomplete recovery, and continued above-average medical expenditures. It is not the growing number of elderly but the increased number of deaths that matters most, since much of the medical expenditures on the elderly are incurred in the last year of life. As the population aged sixty-five and over increases relative to the working population, the burden ·of health care and pension contributions on the latter becomes heavier and heavier, to the point where their net incomes, after paying for health care and pensions, must decline.

Medical technology and particularly public health measures early in this century, followed by the antibiotic revolution and the development of procedures for extending the life of the aged, are responsible for the large increase in the elderly population, beyond the expectations of social security and private pension plans, as well as of Medicare. We have yet to adjust to the fact that life expectancy has passed seventy-five and may soon extend to eighty, as it almost has in Japan. We are not ready for an increase in the maximum life span. It will take most of the twenty-first century to adjust to the large increase in the proportion of the population over sixty-five, to a life expectancy in the low eighties, with a maximum life span around one hundred fifteen. Deliver us from a life expectancy around one hundred, with a maximum attainable life span around one hundred fifty! We are not ready for that. It would be more disruptive than anything since Attila the Hun.

We have been fortunate so far in that the dependency ratio—the ratio of those sixty-five and over plus those under twenty to total population—has been falling, from 89.5 in 1960 to 70.1 in 1990, a result of falling birthrates. This has meant a higher proportion of the population of working age. And an increasing share of the working-age population has participated in the labor force, as the percentage of women in the labor force rose from 37.7 percent in 1960 to 57.9 percent in 1993. Thus, more people have been entering the labor force, working, and paying payroll taxes and insurance premiums. But this trend will soon be ended, if not reversed.

Universal health care coverage is likely to reduce labor-force participation.[8] On the other hand, greater availability and more comprehensive private insurance, perhaps because obtained mainly through employers, increases the labor supply and reduces welfare participation. Dissociation of access to health care from employment, as is true with Medicaid, is likely to have the effect of increased welfare participation and a reduced labor supply. The drop in birthrates, reducing the share of the population under twenty, seems to have ended. And not much further increase in the labor-force participation of women can be expected.

More important is the effect of an aging population. A ten-year increase in average life expectancy achieved through lower infant and child mortality, the type of gain most countries have experienced this century, has consequences radically different from those of the same gain in life expectancy achieved by prolonging the life of those who have already attained retirement age. (Mortality is so low between ages five and fifty that if it were reduced to zero, there would be only a very modest increase in life expectancy.) A life saved in its early years has a much more dramatic effect on population growth because it means an additional seventy or more years of life, and offspring, whereas a life saved for the seventy-year-old means an additional ten or so years, and no offspring. The effects on the dependency ratio—the ratio of non-working-age to working-age population—will have opposite signs. Young lives saved will eventually reduce the dependency ratio; lives saved past retirement age will sharply increase the dependency ratio. A high dependency ratio means lower per capita income compared to a low dependency ratio. A decline in ratio means a speed-up in per capita economic growth, *ceteris paribus*, whereas a rising ratio means a slowdown in economic growth.

Policy Options

Public health measures, including vaccines, were very valuable because they extended useful life many years as well as reduced infant and child mortality dramatically. We have just about adjusted to their impact. Since then, new developments, primarily in medical treatment, antibiotics, other drugs, and new surgical techniques, have further increased life largely in the post-working-age period. And the prospects for further life extension are predominantly among the elderly.

Raising the retirement age to seventy and now setting no upper limits is a step toward countering the effect of higher life expectancy and dependency ratios, but the evidence so far is that its impact may be small. Social security and private pensions are still geared to retirement around age sixty-five; contributions have had to escalate to reflect increased life expectancy (and efforts to postpone work by prolonging schooling). Slowing down the fall in the ratio of working population to those on pensions will not reduce the health care bill; it will only slow down the increase in the burden borne by workers.

Major changes in society will be needed, beginning with steps to raise the retirement age. We must deal with increasing longevity by raising the payroll taxes that finance social security and Medicare or by raising the retirement age for full retirement benefits and possibly the eligible age for Medicare, or a combination of the two. Compulsory retirement (from a particular employer) was initially raised to seventy and has now been abolished altogether, in the hope that many workers would choose to continue to contribute payroll taxes and reduce the number of years during which they would be receiving social security and pension payments. This is not going to work. Eventually the minimum age for full retirement benefits will be increased to sixty-seven, in time to seventy. This has been under discussion for some time, but it will not be done in time to avert further increases in payroll taxes. There are partial alternatives: reduce pension payments by reducing cost-of-living adjustments (which have been overindexed), by eliminating the option of working full-time and collecting full social security benefits starting with age seventy (a double-edged sword, leading some to retire earlier than otherwise, others to forgo full social security and pension benefits until a later age), and reducing Medicare payments by increasing co-payments. Full taxation of social security income is almost on us (already, up to 85 percent of social security income is taxed for some taxpayers), helping recoup pension payments via income tax revenues.

Postponed retirement will not reduce medical spending, it will only persuade or force workers to contribute to pensions, social security, and medical costs for a longer period. If this is not done, payroll taxes and insurance premiums will keep rising, real earnings will keep falling. For a country that through more than two centuries has lived on rising expectations, confirmed by rising incomes, this reversal would be calamitous.

What we are beginning to do is to reduce leisure time over a lifetime in order to pay our medical bills. The large increase in female labor-force participation in the past two decades, from 42.3 percent in 1970 to 57.9 percent in 1993, has accounted for the main reduction in leisure time and increase in payroll tax and insurance premium contributions to date. It has kept take-home incomes per capita from falling. But female labor-force participation is unlikely to increase much further, and male participation has actually declined slightly. If we do not reduce leisure time enough, then we will have to cut spending on other things: housing, clothing, recreation, whatever seems least urgent in our personal budgets.

What must change is the recently invented doctrine of unlimited, unqualified rights. Everyone has a right to food, clothing, and shelter, but no one has a right to caviar, mink coats, and private swimming pools. Everyone has a right to education, but only as much as each individual can productively absorb; no one has the right to a college degree (although social values are tending in that direction, in the process devaluing degrees that were hard earned and well deserved), or a right to attend Harvard (which is impossible). There is no right to plunder the public purse, or others' private purses, for pointless life extension, for high-risk, high-cost procedures with a low probability of payoff. There cannot be a right to organ transplants or admission to the Mayo Clinic as long as the supply falls far short of the demand. Rationing is inevitable. Not everyone can get the best of anything.

Effects on Economic Growth

What the Health Care Financing Administration projections of tax rates and share of GNP do not consider is the negative effect on national economic growth of an increasing share of national economic resources preempted by the health care industry. Without radical change in our health care system, even these alarming projections may prove too conservative. The projections of 18.1 percent in the year 2000 and 32 percent in 2030 assume continued growth unaffected by this massive reallocation of resources to the health industry from more productive activities. They assume no change in the rate of productivity growth and assume that per capita income net of health care spending will grow 0.7 percent a year over the next decades. They do not allow for the impact on growth of a rising share of the GNP spent on health care, especially on health care for the aged. Nor do they consider the rising share of GNP spent on preventive measures, environmental and workplace primarily, which involve considerable investment and nearly all of which lower productivity. These growing expenditures on consumption of health services are bound to reduce savings. Investment in goods and services other than health care and environmental and workplace safety will be adversely affected, as a growing share of reduced savings is switched to research and production for health care and the environment. In sum, the 0.7 percent growth in per capita income, net of health care spending, projected for the next decades implies that there is no relationship between the amount invested or the allocation of investment and productivity gain.

But what about the effect of increased health care spending on labor productivity? What effect? Most of the increase will be for those past retirement age, and in their last year of life. The very modest contribution of medical care to productivity, most of the contribution being from public health, can be obtained by spending perhaps no more than half of what we are spending. The incremental spending contributes nothing; beyond a certain point the amount of iatrogenic illness resulting could reduce productivity. The number of days of restricted activity per capita was lower in 1970 (14.6 days) than in 1992 (16.3 days) or in any of the intervening years. Rick Carlson, fearing that with a continuation of trends as he saw them in 1975, medical spending would eventually reach 10 percent of GNP, recommended diminishing the medical system to half its size.[9] For "medicine cures far less than is generally understood and . . . can cause more ill health than is cured."[10]

There are other negative consequences for living standards of a bloated health care industry. Too many among our best students go to medical school and contribute to the surplus of M.D.s, which makes no contribution to economic growth. On the contrary, apart from the waste of resources implied in educating, training, and creating work for surplus M.D.s, I suspect that, had they gone into other occupations, the economy would have been better off. Most of them end up highly trained biomechanics (no slight to mechanics intended). Frankly, it is a waste of talent. (Similarly, the excessive number of very able students going to law school and practicing law not only adds to the excess supply of lawyers but adversely affects the efficiency of the economy and of the health care industry, instead of the positive contribution they might have made had they gone into productive occupations.)[11] There is no implication that either the practice of medicine or law is unproductive, but the commitment of resources to these activities is far in excess of that needed to attain the best productive contribution.

As long as the cost of extending a life for a year is less than the net income that an individual will produce during the extra year, society as a whole is better off (which is not to say that this is necessarily the best use for the resources employed). But if cost exceeds the resulting additional income, society loses; something else must be sacrificed, whether that something is entertainment or education or housing or investment and growth. What about those who do not earn? Housewives work hard and produce valuable services, although they are not included in the labor force. Retired people have a right to health care within reasonable limits, by analogy to pensions, to both of which they contributed for many years via premiums and taxes. Nevertheless, their increasing consumption of health care not at their own expense reduces the income of others.

Between 1900 and 1950, life expectancy increased by 22.4 years to 69.7, or nearly 50 percent from the 1900 level of 47.3. Medical care as a share of GNP rose at most 2 percentage points to 4.5 percent (we lack a number for

1900). Even acknowledging that most of the increase in life expectancy was attributable to public health measures (sulfa drugs and antibiotics played a role toward the end of this period), it is clear that health care over this period was an investment, in fact a very good investment. Most of the lives saved, furthermore, were of young people, adding decades to their lives. The extra income generated by those whose lives were extended far exceeded the cost of extending them.

From 1950 to 1990, life expectancy grew by 7.6 years, or 10.9 percent, and much of this was in the population sixty-five and over, which rose 3.6 years between 1950 and 1990, or nearly half the gain in total life expectancy. Meanwhile, from 1950 to 1993, the share of GNP devoted to health care rose from 4.5 to 14 percent. Recognizing that much of the gain in life expectancy is attributable to public health measures and lifestyle changes, medical care is no longer a good investment; it is largely consumption, which reduces the income available for consuming other goods and services and the savings and investment needed for continued economic growth. If we look ahead, not much further gain in life expectancy below age sixty is possible; nearly all further gains will be in the seventy-plus and eighty-plus age groups. We might, by 2030, have a life expectancy of eighty-two (the census middle projection for 2050), while spending 32 percent of the GNP on medical care. Clearly a loser.

Health care is not all about life expectancy. What about the quality of life? Are the extra years gained by escalating medical costs good years or miserable years? Is the health and well-being and productivity of the population increasing significantly or not, apart from life expectancy? Days of sick leave are up, not down, but they reflect the greater availability of paid sick leave and a change in attitude of many who regard sick leave as an extension of annual leave, as well as a change from a Spartan to a Milquetoast attitude. There is no convincing evidence, although one assumes there has been some improvement. The development of artificial joints and limbs, laser surgery for eye problems, kidney transplants, and the replacement of coronary arteries and valves have made life much better, but only for a few, primarily older people. For others, Medicare and Medicaid have meant treatment that was beyond their financial reach. For the vast majority, it is doubtful that their health has changed as a result of greater spending on medical care in the past thirty years. It has improved apparently as a result of improved diet and exercise; cholesterol, blood pressure, and heart attacks are down, reducing the need for medical care.

Average real earnings were slightly lower in 1993 than they were in 1970. A time-series study of prime-age adults, starting with ages 22–48, ending ten years older, a period in life when real incomes are expected to rise, found that 21 percent experienced a decline in real incomes during the 1970s, and 33 percent during the 1980s.[12] Another study found that the majority of Americans were worse off in the early 1990s than in the late 1970s, compensating for declining wages by working longer hours and shifting to two incomes per family.[13] We are told that the Consumer Price Index fails to account fully for new products and quality improvements, hence it overstates inflation and understates growth in real earnings. But this understatement also applies to previous decades, when reported real earnings grew substantially. There are many reasons to expect a decline in the rate of growth of earnings, but one of them has to be the fact that we are spending nearly twice as large a share of GNP on health care, leaving less for savings, investment, and productivity growth.

One problem is the protection of living standards from the incursion of the health care industry. With GNP per capita growing slowly, in part slowed down by the diversion of resources to health care, and health care expenditures growing rapidly, the point will be reached in the twenty-first century when living standards cease to rise and begin to decline. (Already, over the past two decades, there has been a decline in real earnings.) This point can be deferred, but only a few years, by postponing retirement, increasing lifetime income even after annual earnings net of health care costs have begun declining.

Unfortunately, because most costs are paid by insurance companies, large employers, and Medicare and Medicaid, most people are not aware of how much of their income goes to health care, or how rapidly this share is increasing, or the cutbacks they are already making in their household budgets in order to pay the health care bill. Some, primarily the young and healthy, are aware of these facts and choose not to buy insurance; they have better uses for their money. Yet we propose to make health insurance universal and compulsory, and perhaps rightly so because we accept a social obligation to provide care to those who need it, whether or not they are covered by insurance, whether or not they can afford to pay for it. But there should be no free riders who can pay the fare. The politically encouraged pretense that the consumer does not pay as long as the direct cost is borne by employers is unfortunate; it removes all limits on the demand for more and more. Health insurance premiums, which were only 6 percent of profits in 1960, grew to 40 percent in 1980.[14] Now they exceed corporate profits, which have averaged around 7 percent of GNP before taxes, under 5 percent after taxes. There has been little change over the past two decades. Clearly the large increase in employer-paid premiums has not come out of profits; it had to come out of wages.

Expenditures on education will continue increasing, especially for higher education, much of which is irrelevant for the economy, and whose growth has already exceeded that needed to sustain economic growth. Too many people are going to college, choosing economically useless majors; consuming, not investing, from a social point of view; and staying too long, in terms of the market for college graduates. If anyone doubts that, look at the jobs many college graduates take, displacing high school graduates who might handle them well enough. Spending will increase to counter the effects of rising costs of exhaustible resources, to reduce environmental pollution, traffic congestion, and other consequences of urbanization and high incomes, setting limits to growth by increasing costs of production.[15] One could go on. Add to these resource-absorbing commitments the indefinite expansion of health care spending.

There have been several attempts to estimate the cost of environmental (EPA) and work safety (OSHA) regulations on growth rates. Edward Denison estimated that they reduced the growth rate by 0.35 percent from 1973 to 1976.[16] As regulations are tightened and additional ones are imposed, not only by the EPA and OSHA, but by FDA regulations for food, drugs, and other medical products and Consumer Product Safety Commission regulations (other federal organizations are concerned with health, but their scope is more limited), the negative impact on growth continues to increase. EPA regulations have diverse objectives, but the main one is improvement in health. The total cost of this other health care "industry" is so widely disseminated that only the roughest estimates can be made of its magnitude, which could be almost of the same order as medical care, and increasing.

Attempting to estimate the impact of increasing medical costs on real incomes would be extremely difficult; to my knowledge no one has attempted it. The basic reason is that the impact of health care costs on growth takes place slowly, incrementally, whereas many environmental policies were imposed rather abruptly, in the late 1960s and early 1970s. One year (1986), gasoline is leaded; the next, no longer; this has immediate effects on octane ratings, costs, prices. One year, power plants and other industries are belching black smoke into the air and our lungs; the next, the plant has converted to cleaner, costlier fuels or introduced stack scrubbers. The costs of electricity, of steel, and of other products are increased immediately, and prices are likely to follow soon enough. The effect on respiratory problems can be detected quickly; but other effects on health take a long time to show a decline. With medical costs, the only analogy is the introduction of Medicare and Medicaid in 1965, which led to a fairly abrupt increase in services, prices, and total medical costs, the largest annual increase on record. Otherwise, costs increase two or three tenths of a percentage point as a share of the GNP each year; only over decades, when the increase cumulates to 5 or 10 percent of the GNP, would one expect a significant impact on growth rates. (Since 1960, the increase has been almost 10 percent of the GNP.)

If increasing the share of GNP allocated to health care were the outcome of free-market choices, no one should object; people choose to sacrifice other luxuries, conveniences, even necessities for more and better health care. But with the growth in third-party payments, there is no real market, much less a free market—a statement to be examined in succeeding chapters. Consumers are not aware of the price they are paying, and many are persuaded that health care is free or nearly free. Resources devoted to environmental and workplace health are the outcome of political decisions, not market choices. The consumer really feels that clean air is a free good. In the absence of a free market and full information, what happens to health care and economic growth as we measure it is not the outcome of consumer preferences.

If health care expenditures are allowed to reach a third of the GNP, while environmental, work safety, and other "nonproductive" expenditures are also growing, standards of living will fall. Even worse, if research and development and investment are reduced in productive areas, the decline in living standards could be substantial. In the long run, these are needed to counteract rising costs of exhaustible resources, diminishing returns resulting from population growth and its concentration in large cities, the rising costs of congestion and pollution. Spending on health will not lower the cost of energy or food or most other goods and services. The problems of disentangling the effect of increased health care costs from numerous other effects on GNP rates of growth over decades appear all but insurmountable. That they have a significant effect is plausible; and that they do not is implausible. We cannot say more.

Notes

1. Sally Burner, Daniel Waldo, and David McKusick, "National Health Care Expenditure Projections through 2030," *Health Care Financing Review* 14, no. 1 (Fall 1992): 1–29.

2. Victor Fuchs, "The Health Sector's Share of the Gross National Product," *Science* 247 (February 2, 1990): 534–38.

3. William Baumol, "Social Wants and Dismal Science: The Curious Case of Climbing Costs of Health and Teaching," C.V. Starr Center for Applied Economics RR #93-20, New York University Department of Economics, May 1993, 24.

4. Edith Rasell, Jared Bernstein, and Kainen Tang, "The Impact of Health Care Financing on Family Budgets," *Challenge* 36, no. 6 (November–December 1993): 12–28.

5. Burner et al., "National Health Care," 6.

6. Ibid., 11.

7. Alan Auerbach, Jagadeesh Gokhale, and Laurence Kotlikoff, "The 1995 Budget and Health Care Reform: A Generational Perspective," *Economic Review*, Federal Reserve Bank of Cleveland, First Quarter 1994, 20–30.

8. Robert Moffit and Barbara Wolfe, "The Effect of the Medicaid Program on Welfare Participation and Labor Supply," *Review of Economics and Statistics* 74 (November 1992): 615–26.

9. Rick Carlson, *The End of Medicine* (New York: Wiley, 1975), 232–40.

10. Ibid., 220.

11. In conjunction with consumer attitudes toward health care and toward environmental safety and preservation that often can only be called unreasonable, the legal profession is responsible for excessive medical care in many cases, and excessive spending toward protecting the environment. Unless major malpractice reform alters its profitability, lawyers will continue to prey on health care, driving up its costs.

12. Stephen Rose, "Declining Family Incomes in the 1980s: New Evidence from Longitudinal Data," *Challenge* 36, no. 6 (November–December 1993): 29–36.

13. Lawrence Mishel and Jared Bernstein, *The State of Working America 1994–95* (Armonk, N.Y.: M.E. Sharpe, 1995).

14. Victor Fuchs, "The Health Sector's Share of the Gross National Product," *Science* 247 (February 2, 1990): 536.

15. Fred Hirsch, *Social Limits to Growth* (Cambridge: Harvard University Press, 1976).

16. Edward Denison, *Accounting for Slower Economic Growth—The United States in the 1970s* (Washington, D.C.: Brookings Institution, 1979), 67–73.

4

Health Insurance Raises Demand and Supply

The various components of health care cost increases are not independent but interact. Because of this, allocating shares of cost increases to particular causes is an oversimplification. But a main culprit of the increased cost of medical care is clearly the growth of third-party payments, including private insurance and various government programs, of which Medicare and Medicaid are the most important. Third-party payments affect all the other culprits.

Insurance coverage increased demand for medical care without concern for price; it allowed increases in fees and prices that would not have been feasible otherwise. The combination of greater demand and higher prices increased the incomes of physicians. Higher incomes attracted more candidates into the medical profession and lured immigrant physicians. The excess supply of physicians resulted in an excess supply of medical services. The larger market at higher fees and prices encouraged research and development of new equipment, drugs, and facilities that improved and expanded the supply of services available and increased spending on advertising, further increasing excess demand. The combination of new treatments and high medical incomes proved an irresistible lure for malpractice lawyers. The multiplicity of insurers raised administrative costs. In the long run insurance coverage may have even affected the age distribution of the population by prolonging lives among the elderly, who are large consumers of medical services.

Health insurance does not lead to these results unaided; a second necessary condition is a fee-for-service system that encourages an oversupply of services at higher prices. A third contributory, although not necessary, condition is technological progress, which provides many new tests, new equipment, new treatments. Without technological progress, third-party payments would have led to large increases in spending, but not to an indefinitely continuing increase. For the effect of insurance per se has little further to go; universal coverage would increase spending slightly, an estimated 4 percent, but once and for all. It is the extension of coverage to new tests, new procedures, new medical problems (newly discovered, or newly made amenable to medical care) that gives health insurance a continued leverage on the other factors raising expenditures.

The Effect of Insurance on Demand for Medical Services

Third-party payments increase the amount of medical services demanded by customers by rendering them insensitive to prices. This increased demand in turn allows physicians to increase the supply of services rendered and to increase their fees and earnings, enticing malpractice lawyers and tempting dissatisfied customers. Drug companies and suppliers of technical equipment are encouraged to increase their research spending, their advertising, prices, and sales simultaneously. Even if drugs are not covered in many insurance contracts, the fact that other medical costs are covered makes the customer more willing to pay high prices for drugs. These effects are exacerbated by tax subsidies for health insurance obtained through employers that lead to the purchase of insurance that is excessive in quantity and distorted in coverage.[1]

What evidence do we have of the key role of insurance (third-party payments) in the increase in health care costs? The proportion of the population insured grew from 50 percent in 1950 to 86 percent in the late 1980s, while the share of GNP going to health also grew, and the prices of medical services rose more rapidly than the Consumer Price Index. But we cannot attribute causation; too many other things also were happening.

The introduction of Medicare and Medicaid in 1965 represented an abrupt and significant increase in insurance coverage. Between 1965 and 1970, the proportion of health care expenditures covered by third parties jumped from 46.6 to 60.5 percent. If we examine the change in share of GNP going to health care services, the increase in prices relative to other consumer prices, and the increase in amount spent on medical services, we note that all three rose more rapidly in the late 1960s and early 1970s than they had risen earlier. Doctors' fees had been rising 3 percent a year, but in 1966 they jumped 8 percent, the greatest rate of increase since 1927; hospital rates rose 16.5 percent, the highest increase in eighteen years.[2] Medicaid's share of third-party payments rose from 7.9 percent in 1970 to 14.6 percent in 1991. Medicare grew almost as fast; its share of third-party payments rose from 11.1 percent in 1970 to 18.2 percent in 1991.[3]

Further evidence consists of numerous studies of consumer reactions to changes in the prices they have to pay. Health insurance lowers prices dramatically. For Medicaid beneficiaries, the price of eligible services is zero. For Medicare eligibles, the price drops by 80 percent of Medicare-approved fees. Most of the numerous studies are not compatible with one another; there is no one number that represents the impact of insurance coverage. Insurance itself varies. Medicaid covers full costs; Medicare covers 80 percent of approved costs. Private insurance policies may or may not have a minimum deductible before they pay; they may or may not have a co-payment, which itself varies. What the studies find is that the increase in demand is sensitive to income; it increases more for low-income than for high-income people. It depends on the drop in price, responding disproportionately to a large drop. It varies with the medical problem, being more sensitive to price for office visits and routine care, less for hospital admissions and acute illness.

Richard Rosett and Lien-fu Huang estimated the overall response to a 20 to 80 percent cut in prices as an increase of 35 to 150 percent of the price reduction.[4] Martin Feldstein estimated the response to price reductions for hospital services to be 112 percent of the price reduction.[5] Gerald Rosenthal's estimates for different types of hospital services ranged from 12 to 97 percent.[6] Most other studies came up with lower estimates. Charles Phelps and Joseph Newhouse found that reducing the coinsurance rate from 25 percent to zero increased demand 28 percent.[7] But the greatest effect was for house calls, office visits, and dentists, least for hospital admissions (which reflect M.D. recommendations following previous customer initiatives). Newhouse and Willard Manning compared full insurance coverage with income-related catastrophic health insurance, 95 percent co-payment, and found that those fully covered spent 50 percent more, including more people using health services and more services per user.[8] But after hospital admission there was no significant difference in spending between the two groups (presumably both having lost any control over their health care). Manning and Newhouse found that catastrophic insurance reduces demand 31 percent compared with first-dollar insurance coverage.[9] The demand is 45 percent higher with no out-of-pocket costs than with 95 percent coinsurance, but most of the decline occurs when coinsurance rises from zero to 25 percent. Daniel Cherkin found that a $5 co-payment reduces office visits for a general physical by 14 percent but has no effect on child immunizations, cancer screening for women, or medication for cardiovascular patients.[10] No two studies are identical, one reason for numerical differences in the findings. But the fact that lower prices increase demand substantially is unquestionable.

Nelda McCall studied the Medicare population and found that the combination of Medicare and private insurance had a large effect on utilization and cost, especially by those who regard themselves as in fair to poor health with first-dollar insurance coverage, who consume 46 percent more medical care than those without supplemental insurance. Those who consider themselves in good health consume no more hospital services (Medicare Part A), and only 9 percent more Medicare Part B if they have supplemental insurance coverage than if they don't.[11] William Cartwright also examined the effect of Medigap insurance coverage, finding that medical expenditures for those judging themselves in poor health rose 14 to 18 percent, depending on the level of Medigap coverage, whereas expenditures rose 48 to 96 percent for those in excellent health, again depending on the level of Medigap coverage.[12] These large increases include greater use of Medicare than in the absence of Medigap coverage. Why these two studies disagree on the relative reactions of those in poor and in good health remains to be explained.

The proportion of the population covered by health insurance leveled off by 1980, yet all three indications of health spending—prices and quantities and total expenditures per capita—kept rising. Clearly third-party coverage is not the only explanation.

The Effect of Insurance on Other Cost Increases

For additional evidence, let us look at some of the other contributors to the increasing cost of medical care. None of them are entirely external to the health care system. A better safety net, including health care coverage for 85 percent of the population, facilitates the breakup of the extended family, which in turn increases the need for outside help in coping with medical and other problems.

The growing elderly population is largely the outcome of new technology, public health as well as medical technology, saving lives and postponing death. The introduction of Medicare and Medicaid in 1965 improved access to medical care for the poor and many of the elderly, contributing to life extension past age sixty-five. This age group uses a disproportionate share of medical resources.

Guaranteed payment, at higher prices, by insurance companies and Medicare and Medicaid assured private firms developing and producing new technologies of a larger and more profitable market, especially for the population age sixty-five and over. In particular, insurance has biased research and development toward innovations that expand capabilities and spending, away from cost-reducing innovations.[13] In combination with the

demand for new technology, both by physicians and their patients, it promoted the introduction of "halfway" technologies that neither prevented nor
cured but greatly increased health care spending (see Chapter 9). The influence of health insurance on the supply and prices for drugs is complicated
and largely indirect. It influences the level and kind of research, the amount
spent on advertising, the competitive pressure to prescribe new drugs, perhaps even the overuse of hospitals relative to outpatient care. FDA requirements for proof of efficacy as well as safety for approval of new drugs,
starting in 1962, increased research and especially testing costs of new
drugs to meet FDA approval, thereby contributing to higher prices and
bringing about a sharp drop in new drug approvals. The longer time required for testing and approval reduces the market life of most drugs, forcing prices up to cover research costs and increasing advertising expenditures to increase or maintain market share. Some new products owe more to
breakthroughs in research than to insurance-supported demand. Most fundamental research was not done by pharmaceutical companies, which rode
piggyback on it, but by the government (NIH) and in universities and foun-
dations largely funded by the NIH, but this may be changing. Prescription
drugs account for only 7 percent of health care costs, but since they are
usually not covered by insurance, except in hospitals, they constitute a
much larger share of out-of-pocket costs, hence the considerable public
concern about drug prices. Were prescription drugs to be more fully covered, and that is the trend today, one could anticipate a rise in price, greater
use, and more pharmaceutical research and development.

The same larger and more assured market increased incomes of physicians
and encouraged continued increase in supply not only by physicians but by
hospitals and other health service organizations and the introduction of expensive new equipment, tests, and procedures. This involved a further shift in the
structure of the industry, from primary care to specialists, and toward hospital-
based treatment, both shifts raising the costs of medical care. It contributed
toward competition among hospitals and clinics for the latest and often very
expensive equipment, toward much duplication, and toward excessive use in
order to cover capital costs. The number of nonpaying patients dropped dramatically, and as long as cost-reimbursement policies prevailed (until 1983 for
Medicare, when it introduced prospective payment based on diagnosis-related
groups, or DRGs), prices and fees could increase rapidly without reducing
demand for medical services. In fact, prices kept right on rising. What fixed
payments for a given diagnosis did is reduce the length of hospital stays and the
number of admissions, reducing the quantity of services rendered, mainly room
and board, but not their prices (see Chapter 5).

So far as litigiousness is concerned, the relations are complex. High incomes of physicians, in large part a consequence of the rapid spread of health insurance, encouraged punitive malpractice suits; so did the shift of medical care from the general practitioner to the specialist and the hospital, both encouraged by health insurance. Malpractice insurance coverage of physicians and hospitals was another inducement. Proliferation of new diagnostic tests and unproven new procedures provided more opportunities for occasional mistakes, for physician obsolescence, and for additional demands for the latest techniques, whether reasonable or not.

Attempts to Reduce the Impact of Insurance on Demand

With health care insurance coverage, no matter how paid, there will always be complaints of delays, denials. As long as customers do not know how much they pay, as long as there is no relationship between what individuals pay in premiums and taxes and the health care they receive, they will always demand more. We are not going to reduce the extent of third-party payments; on the contrary, most propose to extend it to all those not at present covered. How does one dissociate health insurance coverage from inflation of costs? That is the problem.

Customers should be told how much they are paying in terms they cannot ignore. Their payroll statements, their income tax returns, should make that message loud and clear. Ultimately they pay, whatever devices and subterfuges may be used to collect the costs. If they realize this, they may still behave as though health care costs are zero because additional medical services are free or nearly free. But their attitudes toward indefinitely expanding "free" health care could change.

The idea that employers pay or can pay all or most of the cost is absurd, and its propagation among customers is very harmful to the public interest. Total profits of business in a good year are less than the health care bill and soon will be much less. It should be obvious that if employers pay in the first instance, take-home pay will have to fall (or fail to rise as it would have otherwise), prices will have to rise (which amounts to the same thing), and employment fall, or some combination of all three. The alternative, most firms losing money, would be another depression, as in 1933, with 24 percent unemployment. Directly or indirectly, the American worker pays the full cost. One cannot detect the impact of increased employer financing of health insurance over the post–World War II decades on business profits; the costs have been shifted to workers. The difference between no health insurance and health insurance is a mix of price increases, wage cuts, and employment declines. In the long run it makes no difference whether the employer pays all the costs, or the employee pays.

What Kind of Payments?

With 1,500 health insurance companies (this popular number may be exaggerated, but there are many hundreds of players in this field), most of them for-profit, the nonprofit Blue Cross–Blue Shield companies, plus Medicare and Medicaid, there are wide differences in what is insured, who is insured, and insurance payments. In the past, payments were retrospective, reimbursements for whatever physicians and hospitals charged, usually limited to usual and customary fees. This approach was an open invitation to inflation in fees and prices, an invitation rarely rejected. Insurance companies tried two approaches toward limiting their costs by discouraging excessive use of medical facilities by customers for trivial problems that required no treatment or that could reasonably be handled at home. One was the annual deductible, the other was the co-payment. Once the deductible was met, there was no further discouragement of unnecessary demands, whereas the co-payment made the customer think every time. One problem with co-payments that reduce the number of initial visits (after that, there is little difference in medical use between the fully insured and the uninsured) is that "cost sharing reduces inappropriate hospital use but at the price of reducing appropriate use."[14] The customer cannot always distinguish between trivial and serious symptoms. David Mechanic refers to RAND analyses showing that cost sharing inhibited demand in an unselective way.[15] Neither approach deals with the supply side: excess provision of services and procedures.

In 1983 Medicare established a prospective payment system (PPS), based on diagnosis-related groups (DRGs). A hospital would be paid a flat amount based on the classification of the medical problem. For some customers, the hospital would be overpaid; for others, underpaid. There was no adjustment for the initial condition of the patient or the severity of the illness. Some insurance companies began to follow the same practice. As a result, there were sharp reductions in the average hospital stay, but little if any dampening of price increases (it is hard to say what the price increases would have been in the absence of PPS). Some claim that the quantity of services for some customers has been cut too much; they have been kicked out of hospitals prematurely. Physicians and hospitals have some discretion in classifying symptoms and have showed considerable ingenuity in selecting the DRGs with higher payments. In fact, a large proportion of medical services are provided shortly after entry. The main quantity of services reduced consisted of the hospital's hotel and restaurant services. At prices ranging $1,000 and up for a private room, the saving can be considerable. But these are profitable, hence reducing stays leads to price increases elsewhere. The trend away from usual and customary payments to fixed payments that often fall short of full reimbursement tends to reduce demand, although a co-payment known in advance should be more effective than a fixed payment of an unknown share of charges.

There has also been a trend toward fixed payments for specific tests and procedures as well as for office visits. In the case of Medicare, its payments have been close to the customary and reasonable fees, including regional variations, over which it has exercised little control. Medicaid has paid lower amounts, one result being that most M.D.s do not accept Medicaid patients. Private insurance companies and Blue Cross–Blue Shield have also attempted to place lids on the amount of reimbursement for visits, tests, and procedures, but if they have had a restraining effect on prices, it is not apparent. The gap between medical price increases and the rise in the Consumer Price Index was greater in the 1980s than in previous periods.

Starting in 1988, Medicare instituted a new price system, a relative value scale, since revised, relating reimbursements to the cost, time, and difficulty of the service or procedure, which raises prices for general practitioners and sharply reduces them for many specialties, surgeons especially. Whether such a scale will reduce total costs or merely redistribute them depends on the resulting distribution of services rendered between those whose prices rise and those whose prices fall and on the willingness of physicians to accept Medicare patients or perform procedures. It is too early to judge the consequences.

Coverage of Services and Procedures

An ad hoc basis for holding down costs to the insurance company and its subscribers is the practice known as "cherry-picking." Only individuals in good health and with prospects for continued good health are accepted. Alternatively, preexisting conditions likely to lead to considerable medical bills are excluded from coverage. At one time, many companies hesitated to hire anyone over age forty because their health insurance rates would go up. These practices are incompatible with universal coverage and should be on their way out. But there is a problem for those companies with more than their share of high-risk subscribers: their costs and their premiums have to be higher than other companies'. This is the case of the Blue Cross–Blue Shield companies, which are required to accept all comers in return for their tax exemption as nonprofits. Another way of limiting insurance payments is to exclude certain services and procedures. This can be done either on an ad hoc basis or categorically. The practice of requiring a second opinion before approving reimbursement for surgical procedures has become common. There is evidence of decline in grossly overdone procedures such as tonsillectomies and adenoidectomies, but this occurred well before the practice of second opinions became common, largely as a result of publicity on great regional differences in rates, condemnation by the medical profession, and insurance companies' refusal to reimburse. Other procedures long considered to be overused, such as caesarean sections and coronary bypasses, are still greatly overused.

Categorical exclusion of specific services is a more effective way of containing use and cost. Insurance companies offer a variety of policies at different premiums. Some cover prescription drugs, others do not. Some cover general physicals and ordinary office visits, others do not. Most do not cover what is known as "cosmetic" surgery: face lifts, tummy tucks, breast enlargements, liposuction. These are not illnesses, but their correction requires medical care. Radial keratotomy, an operation that corrects nearsightedness without the need for glasses, is usually excluded. Some types of orthopedic surgery, not cosmetic but functional, are in a gray area, covered by some policies, not by others. New, expensive experimental drug treatments, for cancer for instance, are another gray area, covered by some, not by others, in this case because of serious doubts about their effectiveness (concerns about their possibly serious side effects may preclude their prescription) or about their superiority over older and cheaper drugs.

The most problematic exclusion is what could be labeled "behavioral" illness. Smokers pay higher fire insurance premiums; should they have to pay higher premiums for health insurance or be denied coverage? It does not strike the nonsmoker as fair that his or her premium should be higher to cover the costs of someone else's self-inflicted illness. The problem with behavioral illnesses is, first, the difficulty of determining the behavior of millions of people; second, attributing causation. Not every lung cancer victim is a smoker; not every smoker develops lung cancer. And smoking is easy to deal with compared to other behaviors that are correlated with illness. Today the behavioral illness of greatest concern to insurance companies is AIDS because of the very high cost of treatment of associated infections and its present incurability. The high cost drives many victims into poverty and eligibility for Medicaid. Nevertheless, for neither smoking nor AIDS nor any other behavioral illness is there evidence that higher premiums have any effect on their incidence or cost. The problem with exclusion is that the victims are treated anyway and, if not covered by Medicaid or Medicare, for which we pay taxes, or if not covered and unable to pay, end up as a net cost to hospitals that cover them by raising prices on the rest of us. Exclusion only shifts the costs, it does not eliminate them.[16]

Cosmetic surgery and behavioral illnesses both raise the issue of the purpose of health insurance. It is to cover the costs of unknown or unpredictable illness. That is why we are willing to help pay for others' misfortunes and consider ourselves fortunate if others do not have to pay for ours. When health insurance is extended to cover costs that are the likely or certain outcome of willful choices, not only are the costs of insurance raised for all of us, but its moral and psychological support is undermined. When insurance is used to pay for occasional checkups, for the normal, routine ailments that all of us can expect to experience from time to time, that are not expensive and that in many cases do not really require medical care, it is no longer insurance, but prepayment. But, unfortunately, insurance seems headed toward more coverage of behavioral illness and of normal and routine medical care.

What matters most is not the coverage of individuals—universal coverage eventually—but the coverage of procedures, especially surgery, and of tests and drugs. There are two issues here: which procedures and tests are covered, which are not; and to whom is the coverage extended, and for what purposes. Coronary bypasses, caesarean sections, and appendectomies are all covered, but it is clear that too many are performed. What criteria should be met if they are to be reimbursed? For example, blockage of three arteries justifies bypass surgery, but blockage of only one does not, unless it is the left main coronary artery. The condition of the patient must also be a consideration. Existing technologies—psychoactive or psychotherapeutic drugs, the area of addiction generally—are subject to almost indefinite expansion as concepts of unacceptable or undesired behavior and of addiction expand and are redefined as illness (see Chapter 7). Today, nicotine addiction is an officially recognized psychotherapeutic disorder; tomorrow? New and future technologies open up a Pandora's box in terms of who is covered: genetic testing, genetic therapy. Decisions on what procedures and which individuals will be covered by insurance could add hundreds of billions to our annual health care bill.

Notes

1. Mark V. Pauly, "Taxation, Health Insurance, and Market Failure in the Medical Economy," *Journal of Economic Literature* 24 (June 1986): 629–75.

2. Elinor Langer, "AMA: Some Doctors Are in Revolt, but Revolution Is Not in Sight," *Science* 157 (July 21, 1967): 285–88.

3. Sally Burner, Daniel Waldo, and David McKusick, "National Health Care Expenditures Projections through 2020," *Health Care Financing Review* 14, no. 1 (Fall 1992): 1–29; see esp. 26–27.

4. Richard Rosett and Lien-fu Huang, "The Effect of Health Insurance on the Demand for Medical Care," *Journal of Political Economy* 81 (March/April 1973): 281–305.

5. Martin Feldstein, "Hospital Cost Inflation: A Study of Nonprofit Price Dynamics," *American Economic Review* 61 (December 1971): 853–72.

6. Gerald Rosenthal, "Price Elasticity of Demand for Short Term General Hospital Services," in *Empirical Studies in Health Economics—Proceedings of the Second Conference on the Economics of Health,* ed. Herbert Klarman, 101–17 (Baltimore: Johns Hopkins University Press, 1970).

7. Charles Phelps and Joseph Newhouse, "Coinsurance, the Price of Time, and the Demand for Medical Services," *Review of Economics and Statistics* 56 (August 1974): 337–47.

8. Joseph Newhouse, Willard Manning, Carl Morris, et al., "Some Interim Results from a Controlled Trial of Cost-Sharing Health Insurance," *New England Journal of Medicine* 305 (December 17, 1981): 1501–7.

9. Willard Manning, Joseph Newhouse, Naihua Duan, et al., "Health Insurance and the Demand for Medical Care: Evidence from a Randomized Experiment," *American Economic Review* 77 (June 1987): 251–77, esp. 258–59.

10. Daniel Cherkin, Louis Grothaus, and Edward Wagner, "The Effect of Office Visit Copayments on Preventive Care," *Inquiry* 27 (Spring 1990): 24–38.

11. Nelda McCall, Thomas Rice, James Boismier, and Richard West, "Private Health Insurance and Medical Care Utilization: Evidence from the Medicare Population," *Inquiry* 29 (Fall 1991): 276–87.

12. William D. Cartwright, Teh-Wei Hu, and Lien-Fu Huang, "Impact of Varying Medigap Insurance Coverage on the Use of Medical Services of the Elderly," *Applied Economics* 24 (May 1992): 529–39, esp. 538.

13. Deborah Shapley, "National Health Insurance: Will It Promote Costly Technology?" *Science* 186 (November 1, 1974): 423–25. See also John Goddeeris, "Insurance and Incentives for Innovation in Medical Care," *Southern Economic Journal* 51 (October 1984): 530–39.

14. Albert Siu, Frank Sonnenberg, Willard Manning, et al., "Geographic Variation in the Rate of Inappropriate Hospitalization and Influence of Cost Sharing on the Rate," *New England Journal of Medicine* 315 (November 13, 1986): 1256–66.

15. David Mechanic, *Inescapable Decisions—The Imperatives of Health Care Reform* (New Brunswick, N.J., and London: Transaction, 1994), 38.

16. In the case of accidental injury resulting from careless behavior, innocent victims have legal recourse, but most of the awards go to lawyers and expert witnesses, not to the victim. The guilty party may have insurance, and insurance companies discriminate by accident-proneness, on the basis of age, previous records, drinking. But most other behavioral diseases cannot be charged to the individual concerned.

5

The Excess of Physicians and Services

The country can beneficially absorb an unlimited number of individuals trained as physicians.

—Peter Bourne, special assistant on health issues to President Carter

Most M.D.s will practice for thirty or forty years. Thus, whenever a surplus of M.D.s arises, it is likely to remain uncorrected for a very long time. This long lag of supply behind demand is worsened by increasingly narrow specialization. Major technological changes can at any time make specialist knowledge obsolete and greatly reduce the demand for particular sub-specialties and greatly increase the demand for others. (Note the effect of water fluoridation on the demand for dentists, the development of artificial joints on the demand for orthopedic surgeons.) Whereas there is a growing surplus in many specialties, there is a shortage of primary-care physicians, especially general practitioners and family physicians.

It is not easy for a subspecialist to shift to another specialty, nor is it clear that many specialists, even if retrained, would make good general practitioners. The mind frame is different: from procedural skills to cognitive skills to diagnosis, from dealing with specific organs or tissues to coping with diverse human beings.

Subsidies, whether in agriculture or higher education or anywhere else, result in excess supply, even if there is no matching demand: witness agricultural surpluses. But in health care, subsidies also result in excess demand, so that there is no effective constraint on supply. One hears all the time about the debt burden of new medical graduates; one does not hear that medical education once was, and residencies still are, heavily government subsidized. So was the construction of hospitals. Most hospitals and many other facilities are private nonprofits and are therefore tax exempt, as are community facilities. Premiums paid through employers for health insurance are also tax exempt. Medicare and Medicaid are financed exclusively by government.

Too Many Physicians

If there are too many doctors, why is it that they are not lined up to collect their unemployment compensation checks or working short hours or underpaid? Some physicians do work short hours, and the asserted surplus does not apply to every specialty, but there is almost no unemployment, and many if not most doctors work long hours and are overpaid. The reason for the coexistence of a surplus with an apparent shortage in some fields is that the demand for medical services is excessive, and physicians are largely responsible for the excess. Medical care is one area where supply-side economics clearly works; the supply of medical personnel, equipment, facilities, and hospital beds largely determines the demand for them. Once the customer makes the decision to go to a physician, it is the physician who determines what tests, treatments, referrals are made; the customer has very little to say because he knows very little.

We would normally define adequacy as that supply (of physicians, of other medical personnel, facilities, equipment) whose marginal contribution to health is equal to the cost of that contribution. To the well-insured patient, the cost of the additional service is zero or close to it; hence, he is too willing to demand or accept it, even though the social cost (and indirectly his true cost, considering higher premiums and higher taxes) is far from zero. That is one reason doctors find it easy to persuade customers to receive services that should not be performed. Ignorance, of course, is a necessary condition. Since in the health area oversupply does not readily result in unemployment or falling incomes, an alternative indication of excess supply is the relation of the supply of doctors, nurses, and hospital beds to health or mortality. This approach implies a different concept of oversupply: in terms of outcomes, not in terms of demand for medical care. Ultimately one relies on the judgment of experts on the amount of health care that can be usefully provided in a given state of technology, and what human and other resources are required to deliver it. Experts are not always in agreement, but they cannot argue about one measure of outcome: mortality. Large differences in the ratio of M.D.s to population between states and between metropolitan areas are not significantly related to differences in mortality (even adjusting for age and other factors influencing mortality).[1]

Medical inputs, age distribution, and other variables explicitly considered are not the only factors affecting mortality rates, nor are mortality rates adequate indicators of health status. What about health rather than life expectancy? Joseph Newhouse and L.J. Friedlander have used a number of indicators of health status and found the same results: no relation between differences in supply of medical inputs and health.[2]

This approach cannot tell us how many doctors we should have, only that the number of M.D.s required to implement new technologies and exploit existing technologies is much smaller than the number currently practicing medicine.[3] There is no implication that medical care does not contribute to health. But gains in health come about from research and development, not from additional medical practice. During World War II, when 40 percent of physicians were overseas, civilian health improved.[4]

Another indication of oversupply is the growth of advertising, once condemned by the American Medical Association (AMA), which did its best to prevent the customer solicitation practices that are almost universal in competitive industries. Since the Supreme Court ruled in 1982 that doctors and dentists could advertise without interference from their professional associations, advertising has grown. Scanning newspapers from both coasts, I have not found any ads from general practitioners; all the ads were for specialists. In California, some take out full-page newspaper ads and compete in a variety of ways, such as transportation and even meals for customers. These practices seem to be most common for ophthalmologists and ear, nose, and throat specialists, and most of the procedures they advertise are those not usually covered by insurance, particularly radial keratotomy, which allows the customer to see well without using glasses. This is cosmetic surgery, not medical treatment. Although the customer must pay out of pocket, one attribute of the services not mentioned to my knowledge is price. These advertisers are not just young M.D.s trying to enter a crowded market, but experienced and highly regarded specialists. Advertising in the leading eastern newspapers is less flamboyant, again mainly for services not covered or poorly covered by insurance: cosmetic surgery, obesity, substance abuse, psychotherapy. Without adequate independent information for passing judgment on cost and quality of services, all advertising may accomplish is to raise costs and prices.

A final indication of excess supply is the fact that health maintenance organizations (HMOs) use only about half as many M.D.s per capita as the fee-for-service market. One may argue that HMO members are healthier or that they use medical services outside the HMO or that they are underprovided. The difference is just too large to be explained except by an excess supply of M.D.s in the rest of the market.

The belief that there was a shortage of M.D.s long outlived reality. Medical school output grew slowly in the 1950s and 1960s from around 5,000 to around 8,000 a year, then rapidly in the 1970s to around 16,000, where it remains today. In addition, large numbers of foreign-trained M.D.s were admitted to practice. They account for some 20 percent of all M.D.s and 40 percent of residents. The United States is fortunate that it can attract M.D.s from all over the world. But once a foreign-trained M.D. is established in practice here, there is little likelihood that he will leave the country if demand for his specialty declines. Supply adjusts up, not down.

Even after it became apparent that there was no longer a shortage, the training of an excessive number of M.D.s and immigration of foreign M.D.s continued under the mistaken belief that they would locate in areas with doctor "shortages" (rural areas primarily) and specialties in short supply, specifically general practice. Or at least that was the excuse of those responsible for a continuing increase in excess supply. Little of the sort happened; both foreign M.D.s and new domestic graduates flocked to areas and specialties that already had too many doctors; there was some improvement in underserved areas, but at a very high price. Nor is it at all clear that M.D.s from a foreign culture, often speaking heavily accented English and unfamiliar with domestic cultures, would be effective general practitioners (the same is true of psychiatry, which also numbers many foreign medical graduates).

Others were concerned about the coming surplus of doctors by the late 1970s. Joseph Califano, secretary of HEW during the Carter administration, rebutting Carter health adviser Peter Bourne (who stated that more doctors would help control inflation in medical costs), said that each additional doctor increased health care costs by $300,000 a year (more recently estimated at $800,000), in addition to the doctor's own earnings. Califano predicted in 1978 a ratio of 24.2 M.D.s per 100,000 by 1990; he proposed eliminating government subsidies of medical schools, urged medical schools to cut back class size, and opposed hiring more foreign medical graduates.[5]

The Graduate Medical Education Advisory Committee recommended a 17 percent cut in freshman classes. Only a few years earlier, the federal government had been encouraging additional medical schools (which grew from 94 in 1966 to 122 in 1976) and subsidizing enrollments heavily, and the AMA expected the doctor shortage, estimated at 48,000, to get worse.[6]

What has happened in response? Medical school enrollments have not decreased, nor has the inflow of foreign-trained M.D.s. The total number of doctors keeps increasing, from 334,000 in 1970 to 468,000 in 1980 and 615,000 in 1990 and 653,000 in 1992. There is great resistance to cutbacks, not only because of the vested interest of medical schools but because hospitals want a large supply of overworked and underpaid interns and residents to keep their costs down. Yet this very oversupply in time raises medical costs. Hospitals were training 40 percent more residents in 1994 than had graduated; 6,700 were foreign medical graduates.[7]

Most advanced countries have more M.D.s per capita than the United States. Why, then, do we talk about a surplus here? The functions of M.D.s may be different; there are more office visits and phone calls per capita in other advanced countries (and many more house calls) than in the United States. Abroad, a much higher proportion of M.D.s are primary-care physicians. In the United States the ratio of other health care manpower to M.D.s, thirteen to one, is much higher than in most other advanced countries; the division of labor is different from that in Europe or Japan. But ultimately we must define needs not by comparison with anyone else, or even by comparing areas within this country with very different numbers of doctors per capita, but in terms of productive services that can justify their costs.

Since 1970, articles commenting on the excess supply of surgeons have been common. The presence of too many surgeons who performed too many unnecessary operations, in turn generating a shortage of anesthesiologists, was admitted by the AMA as far back as 1972. Evidence of an oversupply of general surgeons was collected twenty-five years ago in the New York metropolitan area. A study of a community hospital found that the average surgical workload was equivalent to 4.3 hernia equivalent operations a week, whereas the desirable workload was judged to be 10.[8] This average load is less than half that in group practices.

So what has happened? The number of general surgeons in 1970 was 18,100; in 1980, 22,400; in 1990, 24,500. Other surgical specialties—orthopedic, plastic, urological, and cardiovascular—have grown dramatically: from 15,900 in 1970 to 36,100 in 1990. The total has nearly doubled, from 34,000 to 60,600.

Specialization

Almost as long as there have been warnings about the coming surplus of M.D.s, there have been complaints about the shortage of general practitioners, including family physicians. Rita Campbell in 1971 noted a developing shortage of general practitioners and a fragmentation of care as specialists came to dominate the practice of medicine. In 1940, only 24 percent of M.D.s were specialists; by 1967, this share had risen to 67 percent. Closed hospital staffs favoring specialists were one reason for the relative decline of the general practitioner.[9] The share of specialists continues to rise slowly, as general practitioners and family physicians, whose average age is higher than that of specialists, retire and are inadequately replaced. Their number today is little more than half what it was in 1949, despite large increases in population, and shows few signs of increasing much. The reduction in the number of medical schools and output of new physicians following the radical reform of medical education prompted by the Flexner Report of 1910, followed by the efforts of the AMA to restrict medical school enrollments before and after World War II, resulted in a decline in the ratio of physicians to population, creating a shortage that afforded them the luxury of specializing in areas of special training, experience, and interest. These conditions are long since past for many specialties. More recently, the sheer number of M.D.s and specialists has promoted subspecialization. What was at first only a division of labor has become a status hierarchy that persists even though many in overstaffed specialties cannot limit their practice to them. There has been what Andrew Abbott calls a downgrading of general practitioners, who are regarded as capable of routine work and not competent to do the work of a specialist (who cannot do that of a different specialist, but this goes unspoken).[10]

The Council on Graduate Medical Education proposes that residencies be limited in number to 110 percent of medical school graduates. The American College of Physicians, the Council on Graduate Medical Education, and the Association of Professors of Medicine agree that 50 percent of new medical school graduates should be in primary care. But the proportion of practicing physicians who are generalists, now 30 percent, is heading toward 15 percent. As recently as 1982, 36 percent of graduating medical students planned to enter family and general practice, internal medicine, or pediatrics; by 1992, just under 15 percent. In 1993 perhaps the trend was reversed, as 19.2 percent made the same choice. The proportion entering surgery held steady at 30 percent, specialties rose from 18 to 32 percent, and support specialties (emergency medicine, pathology, radiology) increased their share from 15 to 24 percent.[11]

The growth of specialization was inevitable. Urbanization of the population created markets that could not exist in rural areas. The development of new drugs, procedures, expensive new equipment, the growth of knowledge, all required specialization and the division of labor. The generalist could not afford all the new equipment, master all the new knowledge, gain the benefit of experience with the new procedures. As previously untreatable conditions became treatable, new specialties arose (oncology, allergy). But this inevitable and desirable specialization has been carried much further in the United States than in other countries, too far, because in addition to the reasons given earlier, specialists came to earn much more than generalists—more than twice as much in many specialties. As the number of specialists grew beyond the needs of the market, even beyond their ability to induce more demand, greater leisure became an added attraction, together with an autonomous work style.[12]

The shrinkage in general practitioners as a share of M.D.s and, in some periods, in actual numbers, and the great expansion in numbers of higher-paid specialists, was associated with the tendency to provide hospital-based rather than office-based services. Hospital-based care grew from some of the same causes—the need of many specialists for expensive equipment requiring many customers to pay for its cost, the impossibility of house calls by a diminishing number of primary-care physicians, accentuated by an insurance system biased against outpatient and office-based treatment, and by subsidies for hospital construction.

Because of the excess supply of many specialties, and the shortage of primary-care physicians, many specialists perform primary-care functions, but at higher prices than those charged by general practitioners. The problem of fee-for-service prices driving medical costs up out of control is one of specialists, not primary-care physicians. Although most surgeons have a workload far below that considered desirable, they report working almost as long as general practitioners. What do they do, other than surgery and related work? Since most of their surgery is in hospitals, they may be engaged in meetings, committees, reviews—and in primary care. Yet it is questionable whether specialists make good general practitioners. It is not only a matter of training and experience, but of mind frame. The specialist tends to have tunnel vision, be procedure oriented, which are not well suited to the cognitive approach, diagnostic orientation of the general practitioner.[13]

The medical profession tends to look down on primary-care generalists (or prizes the higher income of specialists), another reason why their representation in the medical profession continues to decline.[14] I find this strange. Most specialists (I would except psychiatrists) are highly trained biomechanics, whose range of knowledge is often limited, though deep; whose decision-making problems are simple compared to many facing the primary-care physician. Specialists are alienated from one another; they identify with their specialty, not with medicine (less than half of all M.D.s are members of the AMA); they are biotechnicians, with an inflated estimation of the value of their own expertise or procedure and a tendency to overutilize it.[15]

The diagnostic skills of a general practitioner require a vast range of knowledge, constantly changing, intellectual resources, complex decision making. A "unified organism cannot be understood without a unified intellect."[16] Only the generalist has a long-standing relationship and knows the quirks and special characteristics of the customer. In almost every case when specialists are called in, the generalist should be in charge, made fully aware of the specialists' judgments and recommendations. True, one reason primary-care physicians are overburdened and underappreciated is that they handle too many routine complaints—sniffles and cuts—that should be handled by nurses, nurse practitioners, and physician assistants. But regulations, laws, and instinctual defense of territory restrict the range of services provided by non-M.D. medical personnel or require their supervision by M.D.s.

All medical students know, or learn, of the large difference in earnings between the primary-care physician and the specialist. Those who choose primary care anyway undoubtedly have more of the attitude and motivation we have been brought up to expect in physicians—and often have not found. Physicians who choose primary care, especially family and general practitioners, realizing that they would have earned much more as referral specialists, should not be expected to be nearly as profit motivated as those who choose specialization. By and large this is true, although there are many exceptions among younger physicians, mostly driven to pay off large debts accumulated in the course of their medical education.

The physician's traditional mode of solo practice has become increasingly expensive to operate with the great increase in paperwork and administrative costs. A doctor must be familiar with Medicare regulations, perhaps also with Medicaid, and must cope with the forms and regulations of Blue Cross–Blue Shield and numerous insurance companies. Not surprisingly, there is a trend to invest in specialized equipment, to venture into medical procedures where the money is, rather than stick to the cognitive, diagnostic approach that is the primary-care physician's strength. M.D.s who have their own labs and equipment overtest: they order twice as many X-rays and CT scans, 3 times as many MRIs, 4.5 times as many ultrasounds and echocardiographs.[17] It is not practical to return to a 50/50 ratio of primary-care physicians to specialists without a drastic cutback in the use of high-cost, highly specialized equipment. All the testing and diagnostic equipment in many cases drives up specialists' income and widens the gap in earnings between them and general practitioners.

Since only 15 percent of medical school students have been selecting primary-care specialization, the share of M.D.s in primary care (now some 30 percent) will decline steadily until earnings differences are eliminated. Alternatively, more and more registered nurses and nurse practitioners will assume the functions and responsibilities of primary-care physicians (so will underemployed specialists). Nor will the work performed by nurses be limited to substitution for primary-care physician functions. Specially trained nurses and technicians will perform and evaluate more tests and procedures now done mainly by specialists, who are in excess supply and overpriced, which will help to reduce medical costs. Group practice of medicine greatly facilitates the use of nurses for specialized functions now in the hands of physicians.

The ratio of internists and general practitioners to specialists in HMOs is much higher than in the fee-for-service market. As HMOs expand their share of the market, they will bid away general practitioners and internists from the fee-for-service market out of proportion to their hiring of specialists, exacerbating the shortage of the former and the surplus of the latter in the fee-for-service market. Gradually, the huge gap in earnings between generalists and specialists will be reduced, as will the economic incentive for medical students to enter specialties. But without some push, this will take decades. In the meantime, HMOs will continue to be forced to hire too many inexperienced and foreign-trained physicians in their effort to keep costs down. There has to be a better and a quicker way of keeping costs down and equalizing the earnings of generalists and specialists. If specialist incomes were reduced to those of primary-care physicians, we would eventually get specialists with different attitudes.

Earnings

What has happened to the average earnings of surgeons? Of specialists? The shortage of general practitioners was noted even earlier than the surplus of surgeons, with growing complaints and exhortations to increase the share of medical students, interns, and residents in primary care.[18] With a shortage of primary care and a surplus in many specialties, the competitive model beloved by economists predicts that the earnings of specialists should drop, that primary-care physicians should earn more than specialists. What has happened as shortages have worsened for the primary-care physician and surpluses have grown for the specialist? The difference between incomes of surgeons and general practitioners has widened rapidly; surgeons' earnings were around 20 percent higher in the 1960s but began to widen in the 1970s and are now more than twice as high as earnings in primary care (Table 5.1). Earnings of surgeons have been and remain well above the average for all M.D.s. Their income clearly is higher than necessary to elicit an adequate supply; the same is true for most other specialists. Are earnings high enough for general practitioners? Probably so, if there were not ready alternatives at twice their average earnings. Medical specialists in general, not only surgeons, are in excess supply (exceptions include emergency medicine and rehabilitation medicine), their numbers keep on increasing, and so do their earnings.

Table 5.1

Physicians' Earnings

	General and Family Practice	Surgeons	All M.D.s
1965	$ 25,000	$ 32,500	$ 28,960
1970	37,400	45,000	41,500
1980	64,860	97,140	83,700
1992	111,800	244,600	177,400

Source: American Medical Association, *Medical Economics,* various issues.

The argument that high incomes are needed by, and justified by, the high cost of medical schools is circular: the largest cost element in medical schools is faculty salaries. M.D.s need high incomes because M.D.s have high incomes. And the fact that high M.D. incomes drive up costs in hospitals as well as medical schools is a partial explanation for the exploitation of medical students, interns, and residents, who are overworked and underpaid.

The greatest differential between general practitioners and specialists in 1991 is reported here for single-specialty groups.[19]

Family practice	$102,900
Pediatricians	110,500
Internists	114,400
Obstetricians/gynecologists	214,000
General surgeons	254,000
Orthopedic surgeons	327,100
Cardiovascular surgeons	626,000

Most people do not seem to have any idea of medical earnings. A recent survey of public perceptions found that those surveyed thought anesthesiologists and radiologists earned about $100,000 and that a fair income would be $80,000. In fact, at the time of the survey, they earned $221,000 and $229,800 respectively.[20]

Many fields with modest incomes but high entry standards have no trouble attracting more than adequate numbers, even though chances of completion and chances of obtaining suitable subsequent employment are much lower than is the case for medical students. Think of the career opportunities requiring a Ph.D., most of which do not offer alternative compensation higher than that of a university professor. It is hard to believe that a profession dedicated to service, to the preservation and restoration of health, to saving lives, requires the prospect of earnings in excess of $200,000, the *average* for most specialties, to attract qualified candidates—or over $500,000, the *average* for cardiac surgeons. One can claim that the incomes of medical personnel should bear roughly the same relation to professional and managerial earnings as they did when they were set by a functioning market, when payment out of pocket was the dominant form of compensation. That is the way nearly all other prices and earnings are set.

We have already seen that earnings for doctors have risen much more than for other groups, whether we compare M.D. earnings with those of professional and technical workers, with Ph.D.s in health-related fields on university faculties, or with Ph.D.s working with M.D.s at the NIH. We want the amount and distribution of medical care determined by "need," but the income of practitioners set as though third-party payments did not exist. By these standards, medical incomes are much too high. Third-party payments are not the only explanation for medical incomes out of pace with those of other professional and managerial occupations. The restriction on supply of M.D.s in the 1950s and 1960s, by holding down enrollments in medical schools below the numbers needed to replace retiring physicians and reflect a rapidly growing population, may mean that M.D.s were overpaid even before third-party payments became important. Restriction on the acceptance of substitutes for M.D.s (nurse practitioners) and complements of M.D.s (physician assistants) have also contributed to the disproportionate increase in M.D. incomes.

Too Many Services

"[The] high technology interventionist type of medicine practiced in America has lost a sense of priorities and balance. Expensive and sometimes dangerous procedures of unknown efficacy are used promiscuously and often inappropriately while very basic preventive and primary-care services are often unavailable."[21]

Surgery

How is it possible for the ratio of M.D.s to population to have risen as much as it has without forcing down doctors' incomes? There has been a great increase in the rate at which many procedures are performed. One would expect that for new procedures, of course. But for new and old alike, too many surgical procedures have been performed, and in many cases the growth in unnecessary procedures is clear. Surgeons are not the only specialty in excess supply believed to perform an excess volume of services, but surgery is the service most easily examined quantitatively.

Circumstantial evidence that there are too many operations is based on comparison between the United States and other advanced nations for fairly standard procedures such as hysterectomies, caesareans, prostatectomies, and coronary bypasses. Mastectomies and hysterectomies are three times as common in the United States as in the United Kingdom, coronary bypasses six times, surgery per capita twice as frequent.[22] The fact that the United States does twice as much surgery as most advanced countries is not of course evidence that we are doing too much; perhaps they are doing too little. But there is no evidence referring to outcomes that suggests that we are right and they are wrong.

Numerous studies comparing surgical rates regionally within the United States have found large differences in the rates of different procedures.[23] John Wennberg, a major contributor to these studies, asks: "What Rate Is Right?"[24] He finds that differences in morbidity rates between regions cannot account for differences in surgical rates and that there are large differences of opinion among M.D.s about the safety and efficacy of different procedures. He observed that hernia surgery varied little; there was no disagreement on need. But there were no authoritative standards on hysterectomies or prostatectomies, which varied by a factor of four. Lack of authoritative standards on such common procedures could mean that it makes no difference. Presumably, M.D.s in different regions share the same information and experience. The customer should be appalled by the large differences in medical opinion about dangerous procedures that are widely performed. If very large regional differences in surgery rates are often explainable in terms of differences in beliefs about efficacy and safety, one must question the scientific basis of surgery or pause at such a slow rate of diffusion of information among M.D.s.

Other researchers have found that differences in style of medical practice are highly correlated with the ratio of surgeons and hospital beds to population, implying physician-induced demand. Victor Fuchs found that a 10 percent increase in the ratio of surgeons to population is associated with a 3 percent increase in the number of procedures.[25] Each additional surgeon in an area is associated with forty to sixty additional operations a year. The average workload is reduced by 7 percent, but since prices go up, the decline in the average surgeon's income is much less than 7 percent. The low workload indicates a limit on the ability of surgeons to generate additional supply, or perhaps a preference for leisure? The average workload of fee-for-service surgeons is less than half that of surgeons in group practice.[26] The effect is greater for less urgent procedures. Jerry Cromwell and Janet Mitchell found that both fees and utilization rates are higher in surgeon-rich areas, but their elasticities are only one-third of those found by

Fuchs.[27] Thomas Rice and Roberta LaBelle reviewed numerous articles, con as well as pro, and support the view that surplus surgeons induce excess surgery.[28] So do John Holahan and William Scanlon.[29] To clinch the induced-demand hypothesis, the six-fold variation in tonsillectomies disappeared once it was publicized to M.D.s; people did not go to other areas for them.

A RAND study in 1987 found that 64 percent of carotid endarterectomies, 44 percent of coronary bypasses, and 56 percent of pacemaker implants were unjustified or of debatable value.[30] Another study found that 17 percent of coronary angiographies, 17 percent of gastrointestinal endoscopies, and 32 percent of carotid endoarterectomies were clearly inappropriate.[31] As for coronary artery bypass surgery, only 56 percent of these procedures were appropriate, 30 percent were performed for equivocal reasons, and 14 percent were inappropriate.[32]

Since there is much difference of opinion as to the need for surgery, the various studies concluding that a particular percentage of a given procedure should not have been performed at all must be taken with a grain of salt. The precise number we will never know. Nevertheless, I know of no survey that concluded that not enough coronary bypasses or prostatectomies or any surgical procedure (other than perhaps kidney transplants and procedures limited by the supply of donors) are being performed in this country. The ultimate test is outcome measures, which are in short supply. If there are no significant differences in outcome from performing or not performing a procedure that involves risks, the answer is clear: don't.

Additional evidence for the ability of surgeons to increase demand is their response to lower or frozen reimbursements by Medicare and Medicaid. M.D.s responded by increasing the quantity or complexity of services. There was no reduction in expenditures.[33]

Caesarean sections are a notable instance of a large increase in rate of procedures widely believed to be grossly excessive. One in twenty deliveries were by caesarian section in 1968, one in ten in 1974, one in four since 1986. Several hospitals in New York have rates exceeding 30 percent. It is higher for proprietary hospitals and for patients with private insurance coverage. An increase in caesarian sections has been noted when pregnant women become covered by Medicaid, and higher rates are found for insured than for uninsured women.[34] This alone is not evidence of unnecessary sections because some women who really should have had them did not because of inability to pay. It is the actual rates—far in excess of those recommended by expert groups—that suggest greed. The current rate is twice to several times the recommended rate, which need not be greater than 2 to 4 percent, according to nurses and midwives, who may be accused of professional bias.[35] The rate should be somewhat higher in the United States than in most other advanced countries, where it is in single digits, because of the heterogeneity of the American population. The Public Citizens Health Research Group says the optimal rate of caesarians is 12 percent; the Public Health Service target rate is 15 percent.[36] Then why was the rate only 5 percent in 1968? An NIH panel urged fewer caesarians in 1980 when the rate was 15 percent—a tripling in ten years—and noted that 99 percent of those who have one caesarian get another; the task force recommended giving pregnant women a choice and noted that breech presentation caesarians rose from 12 percent in 1970 to 60 percent in 1980.[37]

Several interpretations can be made of this "cesarian scandal," as *Child and Family* described it.[38] One is that the decline in birthrates created an oversupply of obstetricians and threatened to reduce their earnings, and this is how they coped (this oversupply has been reduced as some obstetricians responded to high malpractice insurance costs by withdrawing from delivering babies). Another is that birth came to be redefined as an illness, a pathological event, not to be entrusted to midwives and the like. (In the early 1930s there were 40,000 to 50,000 midwives, but midwifery legislation gradually eliminated most of them, and births moved from home to hospital.) A third interpretation is that obstetricians like to use their skills, not act as midwives. Last, there is a sincere fear of malpractice should anything go wrong, a fear encouraged by the high rate of caesarians.[39] There is some evidence of a positive relationship between malpractice premiums and claim rates and rates of caesarians. It may take all four to account for the enormous increase in the rate of caesarian sections.

With a drop in birthrates, a smaller proportion of births than in the past is to women who have already had one caesarian. Also, the traditional advice, once a caesarian, always a caesarian, no longer holds; the shift in procedure from a vertical to a horizontal incision has greatly reduced the risk of a vaginal birth following a caesarian. The rates should have declined. Instead, they rose.

Another example of supply generating its own demand is based on personal observation, not on statistical analysis. We know that water fluoridation has greatly reduced the rate of cavities and the demand for dental services, especially among the young, whose numbers have also declined, although an aging population will generate additional demand for a somewhat different set of services. Some dental schools have closed, as one would expect. But I have observed another response, which suggest a significant influence of supply on demand: the prevalence of braces. A generation ago, very few children wore braces; now it seems that the majority of children in better-off economic groups "need" braces at some point in their lives.

Tests

Not just surgery, but the number of tests and other procedures has grown rapidly, and seems out of line with other advanced nations. The United States has 2,200 (2,900 since the comparison was made) MRIs to Canada's 22; 919 open-heart centers versus 33; 28,812 hemodialysis units versus 842; 400 lithotriptors versus 11.[40] It has 11,000 mammography units when only 2,000 are needed.[41] An oversupply of expensive equipment leads to an excessive number of tests and procedures (although causation can also run in the other direction) and higher costs. The number of prescriptions far exceeds the number of individuals suffering from the condition for which the drugs are of known value.[42] Hospitals profit from overcharging, so they overprescribe. It is not just too many prescriptions, but a preference for the latest, usually the most expensive drug, on the assumption that it must be the best. TPA, a drug helping open arteries approved by the FDA for those who have had a heart attack, costs ten times as much as streptokinase, is associated with a 14 percent improvement in chances of survival, but a slightly higher risk of stroke.[43] But in this area we are not the only, or even the worst offender. Japan is.

There is a difference in possible explanations for excessive surgery, which is performed by the M.D. paid for it, and excessive tests and especially prescriptions, for which the M.D. is not paid. Tests and prescriptions have always been a convenient way of terminating an office visit, often expected by the patient, but this explanation cannot fully account for their number. In some cases the M.D. may have an interest in the laboratory performing the tests, but this is not a major consideration. The M.D. is more likely to order tests when the equipment is available in his office than when it is not. The hospital is in a different position: it has the equipment and usually the laboratory for most tests, and it sells drugs to patients, profiting in each case.

Half of all health care costs go for tests. The FDA claims that one-third of the 600 million X-rays given annually are unnecessary. Four out of five M.D.s admit ordering many more than needed, for profit and protection. Reduction of the risks of malpractice suits is a partial explanation. The American Medical Association reported that defensive testing cost $40 billion in 1986. And a combination of the technological imperative, try anything new, and the aggressive style of American medicine, try everything, has been given free rein by expanded insurance coverage.

A new way of increasing services and income is the sonogram. This, unlike caesarian sections, is a useful technology already overused. Sonograms are well on the way to becoming standard medical practice for all pregnancies; at least 65 percent of pregnant women get them. As a test or procedure becomes commonplace, it alters the previous standard of practice. M.D.s feel constrained to use such a test or procedure even if they do not feel it justified or are not interested in the extra income it brings. Because the procedure has become expected, failure to use it increases the risk of malpractice complaints and the chances of their success should anything go wrong. In fact, a study of neonatal outcomes could find no significant difference between sonograms and no sonograms (although there might have been a difference had there been no sonograms).[44] No one argues for no sonograms, only for a little more selectivity.

One should distinguish between diagnostic tests and screening tests. The first are given to individuals with symptoms of illness; the second are given to individuals with no symptoms as a means of determining the likelihood that they will come down with a particular illness and deciding whether any measures should be taken to reduce their chances of getting it. The same test may sometimes perform both functions. Screening tests offer the potential of growing in number and cost almost without limit. Sonograms for pregnant women have already been mentioned. An important instance of excessive and costly testing is the mammogram to screen women for breast cancer. (Excessive if medical advice is followed; many women, including those who should, do not get mammograms.) Screening women in their forties does not significantly reduce deaths from breast cancer after seven years. But screening women aged fifty to sixty-nine reduces deaths by one-third. Current guidelines of the National Cancer Institute and the American Cancer Society recommend a mammogram and clinical breast examination for women forty to forty-nine every one or two years; for women over fifty, every year.[45] The AMA, the American Cancer Society, the American College of Obstetricians and Gynecologists, and the National Alliance of Breast Cancer Organizations are all opposed to changing guidelines.[46] But benefits from annual versus biennial screening are minimal. Should mammograms be given annually, biennially, less frequently, to all women over fifty? Should they be given to women over forty? The answer is none of the above. For those whose family history and, eventually, confirmation via genetic testing, indicate a high probability of developing breast cancer—about 5 percent—the answer is mammograms should be given early and often. How often remains an open question. For the rest, they should be given late, and it is not clear with what frequency, but not more often than every two years. Billions of dollars per year could hang in the balance.

The same questions need to be asked, and answered, for many other screening tests: whom, when, how often? But further questions refer to the accuracy of the test itself. False positives may result in unnecessary operations; false negatives, in dangerous neglect.

Louise Russell has recently reviewed the effectiveness of a number of screening tests.[47] Pap smears are almost as effective in reducing deaths from cervical cancer if done every three years than if done annually (91 versus 93 percent), but the American Cancer Society recommends annual tests. False positives are much more frequent than actual cancers. They pose the risk of unnecessary surgery.

The most common tests of healthy individuals are those to test cholesterol levels and blood pressure. Treatment for high levels of either is properly not treatment, since neither constitutes an illness, but prevention, since both are associated with higher risks of heart attacks and strokes. There is overkill in both cases because treatment is likely to begin with levels that in other advanced countries are considered acceptable, and whose added risks are so small that they do not justify the cost or side effects. Twenty-three percent of the population is considered hypertensive. The connection between hypertension and heart attacks and strokes is clear. The benefit of lowering blood pressure with drugs is 40 to 60 percent at best, compared to individuals with normal pressure, but provides full benefit for strokes, as estimated by Jeffrey Cutler and Stephen MacMahon.[48]

In the case of treatment for high cholesterol, there are other reasons to regard it as excessive: the increased risk of heart attacks associated with higher levels of serum cholesterol is quite modest, and there is no credible evidence that lowering cholesterol levels through treatment, which may have to be continued indefinitely, is at all effective. The cholesterol level of 200 to 240, considered in this country as marginally high, is not so regarded in other countries, whose benchmark is likely to be 250 or higher (in the United Kingdom, it is 300). Testing and treatment for high cholesterol with drugs available in the past did not increase life expectancy, except for those who had already suffered a heart attack. Modest reductions in heart attacks were compensated by increases in trauma deaths, for unknown reasons. Even these modest reductions did not take place for adults over fifty-five. It is true that individuals with low natural levels of cholesterol fare better than those with high natural levels, but reducing levels with drugs seems to accomplish nothing.[49]

Victor Gurewich and Murray Mittleman, among others, ask whether Lp(a) or low-density lipoprotein (the component of cholesterol believed to cause plaque) is a risk factor at all.[50] Harlan Krumholz and others find no relation between cholesterol levels and coronary disease mortality or hospitalization for those over seventy years of age.[51] With so little understanding of the role of cholesterol, routine screening cannot be recommended, nor can the national campaign to place millions on expensive and dangerous drugs for the rest of their lives. A few would benefit, but we have no way of knowing who they are; many would be worse off. Thomas Moore summarizes the state of the art: "Diet has hardly any effect on your cholesterol level; the drugs that can lower it often have serious or fatal side effects; and there is no evidence that lowering your cholesterol level will lengthen your life."[52]

Nevertheless, the National Cholesterol Education Program recommends that the entire population be screened for cholesterol and that up to 50 million people take expensive drugs with potentially serious side effects for the rest of their lives. Given the failure of numerous clinical trials to show any benefit (some showed the opposite) from drugs, the recommendations shared by the pharmaceutical industry, medical groups, and government organizations can only be described as intellectually questionable and ethically suspect.

The three tests used to detect prostate cancer are very unreliable; digital detection is likely to come late, whereas ultrasound and PSA (prostate specific antigen) are highly unreliable. Nevertheless, the American Cancer Society recommends annual digital examinations for all men over forty. Individuals whose cancerous prostates are surgically removed live no longer than those who do not have the operation, and many suffer side effects of impotence and incontinence. Most prostate cancers are very slow growing and strike men old enough to die from other causes first. Unreliable indicators of an ineffective procedure should not be used or should be used much more selectively than they are. A few men with fast-growing cancers would gain years of life, but we cannot identify them; a high proportion would be worse off, apart from the cost and risk of the treatment itself.

As to colorectal cancer, there is no conclusive evidence that screening for fecal occult blood reduces mortality. Nevertheless, the guidelines are for annual tests for those over fifty and for sigmoidoscopies every three to five years. The latter can detect up to 55 percent of cancers.[53]

Our concern is with medical need and effectiveness, including medical costs as well as benefits. But financial costs cannot be ignored. Not even mammographies or pap tests are cost saving. There are 11,000 mammography units in the country, whereas only 2,000 are needed; accordingly, fees are too high. Cholesterol testing for everyone aged sixty-five and over every five years and treating those with high cholesterol costs $3 billion to $14 billion a year. Testing everyone twenty years of age and over every five years would cost $6 billion to $67 billion a year. Colorectal cancer screening every five years for those from ages fifty to seventy-five would cost $1 billion a year. If 10 percent of blood tests prove to be false positives, add

$3 billion. PSA screening has not been shown to be effective, but leads to more prostatectomies, which add to costs.[54]

Russell's estimate for screening adults without heart disease for cholesterol and follow-up drugs is $10 billion to $60 billion a year, not counting doctors' visits, in out-of-date prices. Screening all men over fifty for prostate cancer would cost $4 billion. Pap smears cost $1 million per life saved if tested annually, $13,000 if every three years.[55] There has been some progress in revising recommendations to fit the facts, but not enough. The recommendation that women aged thirty-five to thirty-nine get a mammography was discontinued in 1992; recommendations for chest X-rays for smokers and annual sigmoidoscopies for adults were discontinued in 1980.[56]

The screening tests mentioned are only the most commonly performed. The U.S. Preventive Services Task Force recommends another forty-four groups of screening tests. Hundreds of billions of dollars are involved in decisions on what tests to give, who should get them, and how often.

Most tests are no more than 80 percent accurate; one in seven lab tests is wrong or unreliable. Gallbladder X-rays with injected dye are no more than 50 percent accurate, but 200–800 die each year from reactions to the dye. Stress EKG is only 16 to 21 percent accurate in revealing heart troubles in asymptomatic individuals, even less in predicting future heart disease; its false positive rate is 50 percent, and results in four heart attacks per 10,000 tests, and one death.[57] Even mammograms are not fully reliable.[58] Now 50 percent of tests are given in doctors' offices, as 90 percent maintain their own labs, with no control over the training of individuals performing tests in most states. There is a shortage of technicians and a high vacancy rate. Government inspectors began visiting doctors' labs only recently, as a result of a 1988 law.

All procedures, tests, and pharmaceuticals carry some risk. For procedures, unlike drugs and equipment, there is no process or requirement for approval. The control of harmful effects of new drugs lags because of an inadequate postapproval process of evaluation, which depends on the voluntary reports of individual physicians. Steroid drugs can lead to reactivation of tuberculosis; chlorpromazine to Parkinson's disease symptoms; streptomycin to hearing damage; even aspirin to Reye's syndrome. Any intrusion into the body, not just surgery but diagnostic tests that insert instruments and materials into the body—catheters, contrast materials for better imaging, even injections—all involve some risk. Whenever procedures, tests, prescriptions are unnecessary, so are the risks associated with them.

The oversupply of services and procedures is self-reinforcing. Many writers mention iatrogenic illness—illness resulting from treatment—with estimates that from one-fifth to one-third of hospital patients suffer from it. Beyond some point, the more treatment, the more illness.

David Eddy and John Billings find that "some practices are created without knowledge of the actual impact of the practice on health and economic outcomes. . . . The logic appears to be that a practice will be considered appropriate if it *might* have benefit"[59] (without properly considering the effects on those who do not benefit).

Prices

Such a large increase in the amount of services rendered per capita, most notably surgical procedures, would in any other market be accompanied by a fall in average prices. But the reverse has happened; M.D.s have been able to keep increasing their incomes not only by increasing the volume of services per capita (per M.D., the volume has fallen) but by charging higher prices. Areas with the greatest oversupply of surgeons charge prices far above the national average. In a survey of eleven common surgical procedures in five large metropolitan areas, Lauran Neergard found that all these cities, with excess supplies of surgeons, had prices above the national average for all procedures.[60] New York was number one for ten, tied with Los Angeles for one procedure. New York's prices were more than twice the national average for six procedures, nearly twice for two more. It appears that the greater the surplus, the higher the price, another contradiction of the standard economic model. The availability of third-party payments constrains, if it does not preclude, the role of price in limiting excess supply and reducing incomes.

The fact that prices for medical services have increased much more than the Consumer Price Index has already been noted. By itself this fact may not mean a great deal. Were the prices just right thirty years ago? The quality of most of the services has improved, and we lack the ability to adjust for quality improvements. What can be stated is that prices in the United States are much higher than in other advanced countries that share in the quality improvements. The country next door, Canada, has the second highest share of GNP devoted to health, but remains a distant second to the United States. Two articles compare Canadian physician fees with Medicare physician fees, and Medicare physician fees with private insurance fees. Canadian fees overall are 59 percent of Medicare, whereas U.S. private fees are 150 percent of Medicare.[61] (Medicaid fees are 67 percent of Medicare.) That is, U.S. private fees are 250 percent of Canadian fees. Medicare fees, which attempt to approach a relative value scale, are 93 percent of private fees for office visits but only 51 percent for surgery and 46 percent for diagnostic tests.[62] The level of Medicare fees, and to some extent relative fees, are constrained by potential loss of physician participation.

Apart from general price levels and increases, relative prices have been important in encouraging specialization and overuse of procedures. The Harvard relative value scale developed by William Hsiao and associates would award a coronary bypass 30 times the price of an office visit; the actual price is 160 times. Physicians' incomes with the universal use of Medicare's relative value scale as of 1991 would change as follows:[63]

General surgery	−34%
Orthopedic surgery	−42%
Ophthalmology	−43%
Cardiovascular disease	−39%
Internal medicine	−10%
Family practice	+18%

The declines assume that specialists will not prove very ingenious in compensating for price reductions. Even if they are, there should be some decline in average specialist income from Medicare, which might be compensated by increases elsewhere. Unfortunately, the Medicare scale cannot be imposed on the entire health care market. Controlling prices would increase the incentive for demand creation on the part of M.D.s; reducing differentials between specialists and primary-care doctors would increase the incentives for specialists to induce demand relative to primary-care physicians. Participation of M.D.s in Medicare is highly sensitive to Medicare reimbursement levels: a 10 percent change in reimbursement causes a 9.5 percent change in participation.[64]

Given the excess supply of doctors in many specialties, there is a real possibility of increasing the quantity of services to compensate for a decline in their price, thus maintaining incomes. But the high price of services is itself a partial result of the excess supply of specialists, and possible exhaustion of the ability to increase the quantity of services as the number of doctors in a specialty increases. Doctors can increase the demand for services, but only within limits, and these limits may have been approximated in some fields. But it could take decades to reduce the supply of some specialties to the point where an increase in the quantity of services as a response to lower prices is no longer a prospect.

It is only human to resist a substantial decline in one's income, even though it may seem unreasonably high to others. There would be strikes, but what is left of the Hippocratic oath and the excess supply of specialists should render them ineffective. But we need to be wary of the human tendency to make judgments on the basis of extreme examples, "outliers" or "out*liars*." Some new drugs are very expensive, but drugs are a declining share of medical costs. Outrageously expensive "treatment" of a few incurably or terminally ill patients raises slightly but does not drive medical costs.

The excessive number of prescriptions has already been mentioned. Their costs have declined as a share of medical costs, and until a decade ago so did their prices relative to health care prices in general. Since 1985, the trend may have reversed. The price of many drugs, which was expected to fall once their patents ran out and they had to compete with generics, or even before, as they faced me-too competitors, has been raised instead.[65] American drug prices are the highest in the world. Although prescription drugs are less than 7 percent of medical costs, they are about a quarter of out-of-pocket costs because of their limited coverage by insurance. Nevertheless, the excess supply persists, even though much of it—the halfway treatments—makes little contribution to health, and some makes none whatever. Of the 348 new drugs introduced between 1981 and 1988 by the twenty-five largest firms, only 12 were important therapeutic advances; 44 had modest potential for gains; and the rest, says the FDA, which approved them, had little or no potential for advances in treatment.[66] But information about the limited benefits and considerable risks of some drugs is in very short supply. The fact that the pharmaceutical industry spends more than 20 percent of its revenues on promotion—more than it spends on research—is a contributing factor.

With several drugs competing in the same therapeutic market, all advertising does is to drive up prices to cover its cost in many cases. The customer does not comparison shop, and the physician typically does not know the cost of a drug. If there were fewer competing drugs, advertising to increase market share could lower costs through large-scale production. Industry advertising costs would be lower and would not drive up prices. Total industry research and development costs would be lower, and those of individual firms could be spread over a larger output. But often research and development costs are much larger than production costs; thus the effect on prices could be small.

Hospitals

Hospitals are different from doctors because of the hospital's immobility. Population grows in some areas, declines in others. There is migration between regions and states; in large cities, the center loses residents while suburbs grow. Thus new construction in the face of average excess capacity is needed, and much excess capacity is the outcome of changing population patterns. There is a long lag before some hospitals close and others are built. Hospitals need some excess capacity nearly all the time. Demand for hospital beds fluctuates. And there should be facilities to handle such extraordinary events as natural disasters and epidemics.

Hospitals, not just physicians, generate demand for their services. There is a large variation among states in the ratio of hospital beds to population, but limited variation in occupancy rates. The surplus of specialists in turn made it possible for many hospitals to compete with one another in creating and staffing high-cost specialized facilities, such as heart surgery units and kidney dialysis facilities far in excess of need.

The combination of excess overall supply of M.D.s and the major shift toward specialization has meant a shift toward hospital treatment and a rise in health care costs. One study found that a doubling of the ratio of M.D.s to population increased hospital expenses per capita 58 percent; most of this increase represented costs per admission, not number of admissions. The excess costs included greater length of stay (70 percent), greater Medicare reimbursement per beneficiary, and higher prevailing charges of specialist M.D.s. With no change in the number of M.D.s but with twice as many specialists, hospital admissions go up 21 percent; with twice as many surgeons, surgical procedures go up 23 percent. Doubling hospital beds per capita increases admissions by 66 percent, length of stays 14 percent, surgical operations 58 percent.[67] Additional general practitioners significantly reduce and additional specialists significantly increase hospitalization.[68] These studies were made before Medicare implemented its DRG system, which may have affected the reactions.

Most hospitals are private, nonprofit institutions. Hospital administration is under pressure from its medical staff to improve the quality of its services and increase their scope by acquiring expensive equipment. The hospital may feel that such acquisitions are necessary to compete with other hospitals for physicians and patients.[69] The result is duplication of services and facilities, excess capacity, a greater quantity and higher quality and presumably higher cost than would prevail in a private, for-profit market. Duplication of services and facilities is not motivated by the desire to provide better access. The resulting underuse (or unnecessary use) raises prices and total expenditures.

Although much of the overcapitalization and overstaffing of hospitals is intended to improve the quality of services, some excess capacity may have adverse consequences on the quality of treatment. Open-heart surgery requires a team of specialists, whose proficiency depends on frequent performance. As a rule of thumb, a team must perform a minimum of 100 procedures a year to maintain its skill as a team and as individuals on that

Table 5.2

Community Hospital Utilization

	Beds per 1,000	Occupancy (%)	Admissions per 1,000	Average Stay (days)	Employment per Patient
1960	3.6	74.7	136	7.6	226
1970	4.3	77.3	152	8.0	265
1980	4.5	75.2	159	7.3	334
1990	3.8	66.8	125	6.4	417
1992	3.6	65.6	122	6.2	436

Source: American Hospital Association, *Hospital Statistics* (Chicago: AHA, 1994 and earlier years).

team. The result is reduced mortality and improved quality.[70] Yet many hospitals perform only a small fraction of the number of procedures required to develop and maintain skills. The fact that so many hospitals are prepared to perform only a few procedures of the type where experience and skill is important for the lives of patients means that fewer hospitals are able to perform enough procedures to attain and maintain these skill levels, precluding the attainment of the full advantages of specialization.

Albert Siu and others examined the geographical variation in rates of hospitalization and lengths of hospital stays.[71] They found that 23 percent of admissions and one-third of hospital days were inappropriate; another 17 percent of admissions were avoidable via ambulatory surgery. There was little difference between patients with full coverage and those with cost sharing, although they found that cost sharing reduced both appropriate and inappropriate hospital utilization. A study of Medicare and Medicaid admissions found that 19 percent of admissions and 27 percent of hospital days were inappropriate.[72]

Efforts to limit increases in health care costs have been concentrated on hospitals, which account for nearly 40 percent of the total costs and nearly all the high-cost procedures. They have had some success, reducing hospital costs as a share of total costs, but much of this reduction has been countered by greater use of outpatient care and nursing homes.

The number of hospitals has been declining slowly, but the number of hospital beds per capita has fallen by half. Nevertheless, the occupancy rate (the percentage of beds occupied) has also fallen, particularly in 1984, the first year in which Medicare applied its new system of reimbursement, a flat amount per diagnostic classification. Hospital admission rates rose from

136 per 1,000 in 1960 to a high of 159 in 1980 but have declined since to 125 in 1990 and 122 in 1992. The average stay, which was 8 days in 1970, has dropped steadily to 7.3 in 1980, then abruptly to 6.5 in 1985, no doubt a response to efforts by Medicare in particular to restrain the rise in costs by setting specific reimbursements for DRGs. It has declined little since, to 6.4 days in 1990 and 6.2 days in 1992 (Table 5.2). Since the early 1980s, hospital-bed days have declined 30 percent, through a combination of lower admission rates and fewer days per admission. Under the formerly prevailing practice of reimbursement by insurance companies based on "usual, customary and reasonable" fees, there was an incentive for fees to rise. Unfortunately, the pressures to contain costs have not kept fees from rising, only quantity of services. Despite the reduced admission rates and average stays, hospital employment during the 1980s increased from 2.75 million in 1980, declined slightly during the mid-1980s, then rose again to 3.56 million in 1990, and by 1993 to 3.82 million. Thus hospital personnel per occupied bed has risen from 1.14 in 1960 to 1.96 in 1970 to 3.7 today.

As a result of the DRG reform instituted in 1983, hospitals are competing more vigorously than ever for patients. They must either increase volume or cut costs. They have added outpatient clinics, some have even introduced house calls, and seek to lure M.D.s with large practices or admission rates. The average of 3.7 full-time employees per occupied bed suggests that empty beds are not the only problem.

One still hears complaints about unnecessary hospitalization. One hears about hospital admissions that should have been treated on an outpatient basis. There will always be some unnecessary hospitalizations, and some not admitted who should have been. It's a question of how many. Beliefs tend to lag well after facts. Determined efforts to contain costs have been under way for nearly two decades. They have had substantial success in reducing quantity of service: the rate of hospital admissions is down, the average length of hospital stays is way down. But the share of hospitals in health care costs has not declined appreciably. A disproportionate share of costs is incurred in the first day of admission, so fewer admissions, not shorter stays, should have had the major impact in reducing hospital costs. The main cost saving from shorter stays is the room charge. And lower admissions, while reducing hospital costs, may not be a net reduction in medical costs, since they are associated with more outpatient care and more nursing home admissions.

The main evidence that there are still too many admissions is the experience of HMOs, which have as much as a 40 percent lower rate of admissions than fee-for-service care. There are questions whether the HMO rates may be too low, and whether HMO users may not be lower in health care needs than the rest of the population. Another kind of evidence is the substantial interstate difference in length of stay for identical conditions, assuming that the shorter stays are not too short. A third indication that more can be done is the high correlation between number of hospital beds and hospital utilization, which is a product of admission rates and average length of stay, suggesting that supply is still creating its own demand.

There has been a surplus of hospital beds for quite a few years, which appears to be still growing. The number of hospital-bed days per capita in the United States in 1990, 1.2, is less than half of what it was in 1960 (2.8), and much lower than in other OECD countries except for the poorest: Portugal, Spain, Greece, and Turkey. Average lengths of stay were much shorter than in other OECD countries, except Denmark, slightly lower, and Turkey, slightly higher.[73] Since the United States has far fewer beds per capita than other industrial nations, less than half as many as France or Germany, lower even than the United Kingdom, a much lower rate of hospital admissions, and much shorter average stays, it is not clear that hospitals are overutilized. At the same time that we have lower admission rates and shorter stays, we greatly outperform other advanced nations in most surgical procedures that require hospitalization. Too many are performed. Reducing the number of surgical procedures would reduce admissions and in many cases the length of stay (normal deliveries versus caesarian sections, for instance).

Then why are American hospitals facing low occupancy, while critics complain about their overuse? One cannot compare foreign and American hospitals directly; their roles differ between countries. Individuals may be admitted elsewhere who in this country would be directed to outpatient facilities or nursing homes. The number of hospital personnel per occupied bed in the United States is much higher than in other industrial countries. Looking at specific illnesses and procedures, the United States has the shortest hospital stay, often by a wide margin, for a wide variety of illnesses, in spite of the fact that other countries are all much more successful in containing their health care costs than the United States. These facts suggest that the United States is placing too much stress on reducing quantity, because it has been unable, or unwilling, to reduce excessive prices and pay.

If policies reducing admissions and length of stays have had much effect on prices, it is not apparent in overall price trends, which were higher in the 1980s than in earlier periods. The dominance of the fee-for-service system limits the ability of Medicare, insurance companies, and hospitals to influence prices. Nor is it clear that doctor-dominated institutions such as non-profit hospitals, or even Blue Cross–Blue Shield, have much interest in holding down increases in fees, much less reducing them. Freedom to raise fees gives hospitals the flexibility to shift costs.

If we do not succeed in reducing prices (or their rate of increase, as the case may be), we face the prospect that an unbalanced stress on reducing quantity of services and procedures could go too far, in particular because DRG compensation makes inadequate allowance for the initial condition of the patient or for the severity or complexity of the illness or procedure. In fact, such a stress makes the M.D. more prone to raise fees, as the only way of maintaining or increasing earnings. If we could restrain prices, there would be less incentive for hospitals to reduce the quantity of services rendered, inasmuch as quantity would then be the preferred, if not the only, means of preserving or increasing earnings.

And then there are the veterans' hospitals—171 of them, costing $17 billion a year, most of them of poor quality, most of them scampering for patients to fill their beds. They should be closed. There may be a few areas where the presence of a veterans' hospital could preclude the need to build another, if this hospital were open to the general public; but then it would cease to be a veterans' hospital. Veterans' hospitals, like the Rural Electrification Administration, are evidence that bureaucracies live forever even though their job is done.

Notes

1. Richard Auster, Irving Leveson, and Deborah Sarachek, "The Production of Health: An Exploratory Study," *Journal of Human Resources* 4 (Fall 1969): 411–36. See also Charles T. Stewart, Jr., "Distribution of Medical Inputs across Standard Metropolitan Statistical Areas and Implications for Health," in *Advances in Health Economics and Health Services Research*, ed. Richard Scheffler and Louis Rossiter, 191–220 (Greenwich, Conn.: JAI Press, 1982).

2. Joseph Newhouse and L.J. Friedlander, "The Relationship between Medical Resources and Measures of Health: Some Additional Evidence," *Journal of Human Resources* 15 (Spring 1980): 200–218.

3. Rick Carlson, *The End of Medicine* (New York: Wiley, 1975), 232–40.

4. Rosemary Stevens, *American Medicine and the Public Interest* (New Haven, Conn.: Yale University Press, 1971), 354.

5. R. Jeffrey Smith, "Carter Attempt to Limit Doctor Supply Faces Tough Going in Congress," *Science* 203 (February 16, 1979): 122. William Metz, "Califano to Medical Schools: Cut Back Class Size," *Science* 202 (November 17, 1978): 726.

6. Richard Lyons, "AMA Expects the Doctor Shortage to Get Worse," *Washington Evening Star and Daily News,* November 23, 1972, B5.

7. David Kindig, "Specialist Glut, Generalist Shortage," *Washington Post,* September 7, 1994, A21.

8. Edward F.X. Hughes, Victor Fuchs, John Jacoby, and Eugene Lewit, "Surgical Workloads in a Community Practice," *Surgery* 71 (March 1972): 315–27.

9. Rita Ricardo Campbell, *Economics of Health and Public Policy* (Washington, D.C.: American Enterprise Institute, 1971), 11, 95.

10. Andrew Abbott, *The System of Professions: An Essay on the Division of Expert Labor* (Chicago: University of Chicago Press, 1988), 125–27. More recently, the sheer number of M.D.s and specialists has promoted subspecialization, as predicted by Durkheim. See George Simpson, *Emile Durkheim on the Division of Labor in Society* (New York: MacMillan, 1933), 257–62. Durkheim attributes specialization to numbers, population density, urbanization, and improved transportation and communication, basically to market size.

11. Daniel Q. Haney, "Medical Generalists 'Get No Respect,'" *Washington Times,* June 9, 1993, E3.

12. Niccie McKay, "The Economic Determinants of Specialty Choice by Medical Residents," *Journal of Health Economics* 9 (November 1990): 335–57. See also Michael Rosenthal, James Diamond, Howard Rabinowitz, et al., "Influence of Income, Hours Worked and Loan Repayment on Medical Students' Decision to Pursue a Primary Care Career," *Journal of the American Medical Association* 271 (March 23/30, 1994): 914–17.

13. Anita Slomski, "Can Specialists Really Turn into Generalists?" *Medical Economics* 70 (December 13, 1993): 127–31.

14. Haney, "Medical Generalists 'Get No Respect.'"

15. Edmund Pellegrino, "The Sociocultural Impact of Twentieth Century Therapeutics," in *The Therapeutic Revolution—Essays in the Social History of American Medicine,* ed. Morris Vogel and Charles Rosenberg, 245–66 (Philadelphia: University of Pennsylvania Press, 1979).

16. Scott Buchanan, *The Doctrine of Signatures—a Defense of Theory in Medicine,* 2nd ed., ed. Peter Mayock, Jr. (Urbana and Chicago: University of Illinois Press, 1991), xxi.

17. Spencer Rich, "Doctors Who Own Equipment Order More Tests, Study Shows," *Washington Post,* April 15, 1994, A14.

18. Jay Nelson Tuck, "New Classes for the Student Doctor," *New York Times,* November 14, 1971, E10.

19. Anita Slomski, "Groups Dangle Big Salaries—but for How Long?" *Medical Economics* 70 (February 8, 1993): 52.

20. Kathleen Day, "In Health Care, Pay Outpaces Perception," *Washington Post,* March 31, 1993, F1.

21. David Mechanic, *Inescapable Decisions—the Imperatives of Health Reform* (New Brunswick, N.J., and London: Transactions, 1994), xi.

22. Lynn Payer, *Medicine and Culture* (New York: Holt, 1988).

23. John Wennberg and Alan Gittelsohn, "Variations in Medical Care among Small Areas," *Scientific American* 246, no. 4 (April 1982): 120–34. The entire issue of *Health Affairs* for Summer 1984 is devoted to this subject.

24. John Wennberg, "Which Rate Is Right?" *New England Journal of Medicine* 314 (January 30, 1986): 310–11.

25. Victor Fuchs, "The Supply of Surgeons and the Demand for Operations," *Journal of Human Resources* Supplement 13 (1978): 35–56, esp. 54.

26. Victor Fuchs, *The Health Economy* (Cambridge, Mass.: Harvard University Press, 1986): 129.

27. Jerry Cromwell and Janet Mitchell, "Physician-Induced Demand for Surgery," *Journal of Health Economics* 5 (December 1986): 293–313.

28. Thomas Rice and Roberta Labelle, "Do Physicians Induce Demand for Medical Services?" *Journal of Health Politics, Policy and Law* 14 (Fall 1989): 587–600.

29. John Holahan and William Scanlon, *Price Controls, Physician Fees and Physician Incomes from Medicare and Medicaid* (Washington, D.C.: Urban Institute, 1978).

30. "Fallible Doctors," *Economist,* December 17, 1988, 19–21.

31. Mark Chassin, Jacqueline Kosecoff, R.E. Park, et al., "Does Inappropriate Use Explain Geographic Variations in the Use of Health Care Services?" *Journal of the American Medical Association* 258 (November 13, 1987): 2533–37.

32. Constance Monroe Winslow, Jacqueline Kosecoff, Mark Chassin, et al., "The Appropriateness of Performing Coronary Bypass Surgery," *Journal of the American Medical Association* 260 (July 22–29, 1988): 505–9. The RAND Corporation has produced a large number of reports on the same subject.

33. Jon Gobel and Thomas Rice, "Reducing Public Expenditures for Physician Services: The Price of Paying Less," *Journal of Health Politics, Policy and Law* 9 (Winter 1985): 595–609.

34. Jennifer Haas, Sven Udvarhelyi, and Arnold Epstein, "The Effect of Health Coverage for Uninsured Pregnant Women on Maternal Health and the Use of Caesarian Section," *Journal of the American Medical Association* 270 (July 7, 1993): 61–64.

35. *Newsletter of the International Cesarian Awareness Network,* New York City chapter, Winter 1994.

36. David Brown, "Twenty-Year Rise in Caesarian Deliveries Appears to Have Stopped," *Washington Post,* May 19, 1994, A26.

37. Gina Kolata, "NIH Panel Urges Fewer Caesarian Births," *Science* 210 (October 10, 1980): 176–77.

38. American Public Health Association, "Reducing Cesarians," *Child and Family* 21, no. 3 (1993): 210–14.

39. A. Russell Localio, Ann Lawthers, Joan Bengtson, et al., "Relation between Malpractice Claims and Caesarian Delivery," *Journal of the American Medical Association* 269 (January 20, 1993): 366–73.

40. David Azevedo, "Canada: The Truth about Queues," *Medical Economics* 70 (May 24, 1993): 167–83.

41. Ken Terry, "How Much Preventive Care Can We Afford?" *Medical Economics* 70 (August 23, 1993): 124–36, esp. 128.

42. Charlotte Muller, "The Overmedicated Society," *Science* 176 (May 5, 1972): 488–92.

43. "Wider Use of Heart Drug Endorsed by FDA Panel," *Washington Post/Health,* June 14, 1994, 5.

44. Bernard Ewigwam, James Crane, Fredric Frigoletto, et al., "Effect of Prenatal Ultrasound Screening on Perinatal Outcome," *New England Journal of Medicine* 329 (September 16, 1993): 821–27.

45. Christine Russell, "Mammogram Review—NIH to Reassess Guidelines," *Washington Post/Health,* March 23, 1993, 9.

46. Christine Russell, "Mammography Guidelines Come under Scrutiny," *Washington Post/Health,* November 23, 1993, 10.

47. Louise Russell, *Educated Guesses—Making Policy about Medical Screening Tests* (Berkeley: University of California Press, 1994).

48. Louise Russell, *Evaluating Preventive Care—a Report on a Workshop* (Washington, D.C.: Brookings Institution, 1987): 16.

49. Thomas Moore, *Lifespan* (New York: Simon and Schuster, 1993): 184–204.

50. Victor Gurewich and Murray Mittleman, "Lipoprotein(a) in Coronary Heart Disease—Is It a Risk Factor at All?" *Journal of the American Medical Association* 271 (April 6, 1994): 1025–26.

51. Harlan Krumholz, Teresa Seeman, Susan Merrill, et al., "Lack of Association between Cholesterol and Coronary Heart Disease and Morbidity and All-Cause Mortality in Persons Older Than 70 Years," *Journal of the American Medical Association* 272 (November 2, 1994): 1335–40.

52. Thomas J. Moore, "The Cholesterol Myth," *Atlantic Monthly,* September 1989, 37–70, esp. 37.

53. Jack Mandel, John Bond, Timothy Church, et al., "Reducing Mortality from Colorectal Cancer by Screening for Fecal Occult Blood," *New England Journal of Medicine* 328 (May 13, 1993): 1365–71. David Ahlquist, Charles Moertel, and Douglas McGill, "Screening for Colorectal Cancer," *New England Journal of Medicine* 329 (October 21, 1993): 1351.

54. Terry, "How Much Preventive Care Can We Afford?"

55. Russell, *Educated Guesses,* 78–82.

56. Robert Badgett, "Screening for Prostate Cancer," *New England Journal of Medicine* 330 (January 13, 1994): 220. See also Harold Sox, Jr., "Preventive Health Services in Adults," *New England Journal of Medicine* 330 (June 24, 1994): 1589–95, for some current recommendations of the American College of Physicians and the U.S. Preventive Services Task Force, and comments.

57. Cathey Pinckney and Edward Pinckney, "Needless Medical Tests—a $40 Billion Boondoggle," *Washington Post,* August 16, 1987, D1.

58. Joann Elmore, Carolyn Wells, Carol Lee, et al., "Variability in Radiologists' Interpretations of Mammograms," *New England Journal of Medicine* 331 (December 1, 1994): 1493–99.

59. David Eddy and John Billings, "The Quality of Medical Evidence," *Health Affairs* 7, no. 1 (1988): 19–32, esp. 27.

60. Lauran Neergard, "Patients Offered Level Playing Field in Buying Health Care." *Washington Times,* November 27, 1993, D5, D8.

61. Pete Welch, Steven Katz, and Stephen Zuckerman, "Physicians Fee Levels: Medicare versus Canada," *Health Care Financing Review* 14, no. 3 (Spring 1993): 41–54.

62. Mark Miller, Stephen Zuckerman, and Michael Gates, "How Do Medicare Physician Fees Compare with Private Payers?" *Health Care Financing Review* 14, no. 3 (Spring 1993): 25–39.

63. Paul Ginsburg, "Why Your Income Is Where It Is Now and Where It's Going," *Medical Economics* 71 (May 23, 1994): 60–69.

64. Janet Mitchell, Margo Rosenbach, Jerry Cromwell, et al., "To Sign or Not to Sign: Physician Participation in Medicare, 1984," *Health Care Financing Review* 10, no. 1 (Fall 1988): 17–28.

65. Don Colburn, "Drug Prices: What's Up?" *Washington Post/Health,* December 15, 1992, 8–13.

66. F. Roy Vagelos, "Are Prescription Drug Prices High?" *Science* 252 (May 24, 1991): 1080–84.

67. Karen Davis, "Physician Supply and Health Care Costs," in *The Coming Physician Surplus—in Search of a Policy,* ed. Eli Ginsburg and Miriam Ostrow, 37–48 (Totowa, N.J.: Rowman and Allanheld, 1984).

68. Martin Feldstein, "Hospital Cost Inflation: A Study of Nonprofit Price Dynamics," *American Economic Review* 61 (December 1971): 864.

69. *American Economic Association Papers and Proceedings* 77 (May 1987): 257–62; Maw Lin Lee, "A Conspicuous Production Theory of Hospital Behavior," *Southern Economic Journal* 38 (July 1971): 48–58; Susan Parker, "Competing for Patients," *Washington Post/Health,* 5 June 1985, 12, 13; Spencer Rich, "Hospitals Are Competing for Patients," *Washington Post,* March 11, 1984, A1, A5.

70. James Jollis, Eric Peterson, Elizabeth DeLong, et al., "The Relation between the Volume of Coronary Angioplasty Procedures at Hospitals Treating Medicare Beneficiaries and Short-Term Mortality," *New England Journal of Medicine* 331 (December 15, 1994): 1625–29.

71. Albert Siu, Frank Sonnenberg, Willard Manning, et al., "Geographic Variation in Rate of Inappropriate Hospitalization and Influence of Cost Sharing on the Rate," *New England Journal of Medicine* 315 (November 13, 1986): 1256–66.

72. Joseph Restuccia, Paul Gertman, Susan Dayno, et al., "The Appropriateness of Hospital Use," *Health Affairs* 3, no. 2 (Summer 1984): 30–38.

73. George Schieber, Jean-Pierre Poullier, and Leslie Grunwald, "U.S. Health Expenditure Performance: An International Comparison," *Health Care Financing Review* 13, no. 4 (Summer 1992): 1–87; see also 24.

6

The Medicalization of Health

Supply Creates Demand

Rick Carlson, in his much-praised *The End of Medicine,* written in 1975, prescribed cutting the number of physicians in half and shifting the distribution heavily toward primary care.[1] The resources released could make a greater contribution to health and life in other employment. He must be surprised to note that in fact the number of physicians has almost doubled, and has further skewed toward specialists, and that the health care industry has far surpassed his feared 10 percent of GNP. How did this come about? We have reviewed the facts about the vast expansion of supply. But how did everyone manage to keep busy?

The medical profession has succeeded so far in increasing the demand for its services to such an extent that a near-doubling of the ratio of doctors to population since 1960 has not resulted in a surplus of M.D.s in general or in almost any specialty (in the sense that incomes fall, or prices fall, or M.D.s are unemployed, although many specialists have more leisure time than they should have). This was accomplished in part, as previously indicated, by overtesting and overtreatment. Comparison of rates in the United States with rates in other advanced and wealthy countries gives an indication of oversupply in many services: caesarian sections, coronary bypasses, surgical rates in general, therapy for high serum cholesterol, high blood pressure treatment, and a wide variety of diagnostic and screening tests. For that matter, comparisons of rates in different regions within the United States give the same indication: the more surgeons per capita, the more surgical procedures; the more hospital beds, the higher the rate of hospital admission relative to populations. We are not suggesting that low rates are necessarily appropriate and that high rates constitute overuse. But the lack of evidence that outcomes are better in the high-rate areas and countries does suggest overuse.

In addition to extending treatment in the direction of marginal or questionable need or benefit, but far from trivial cost or risk, the health care industry has extended its boundaries, defining conditions as illnesses that formerly were not so considered and colonizing new areas for testing and treatment. Important areas are a vastly expanded concept of mental illness, including drug and alcohol abuse, and, just getting started, genetic screening and, already at the experimental stage, genetic therapy.

It is not easy to draw a clear line between more services within given boundaries and the extension of boundaries. At one time, screening for cholesterol was new, now it is almost universally done. Already mentioned is the fact that in other countries treatment for serum cholesterol is rarely considered until it exceeds 250 (300 in the United Kingdom), whereas in the United States some M.D.s and customers start worrying if it exceeds 200, which is below the national average, but described as "marginally high." Treatment for high blood pressure also is initiated and pursued aggressively at lower levels here than abroad. There is a tendency to consider normal pregnancy and birth, along with old age, as illnesses. What is overuse of existing tests and treatments? What is an extension of the boundaries of medical care?

As long as physicians and hospitals are reimbursed on a fee-for-service basis, they will have a strong interest both in oversupplying services and in extending the boundaries of medical care. The only way to eliminate this bias is to sever the relationship between earnings and amount of services rendered—to place physicians on a salary. Hospital management might still retain a bias, but not the M.D. who is the individual decision maker. As evidence, look at Japan. Japanese M.D.s sell drugs directly to the customer. The result is that Japan spends a much larger proportion of its medical bill on drugs than any other country and that much of the earnings of primary-care physicians come from profits on the sale of drugs. They are drug pushers. More important than method of payment is the large and growing surplus of specialists. This surplus leads to the development of subspecialties and new specialties, in the process inventing new illnesses and treatments.

What Is Health, What Is Illness?

Accepting a nearly universal consensus that all Americans should have health care insurance and receive health care, several questions remain to be answered: What is health? What is medical care? How much is adequate? Implicitly, what should be reimbursed by insurance and what should not?

Many services performed by M.D.s in a health care setting have nothing to do with health. Therefore they should not be covered by insurance or counted as medical costs. Another way of putting it is that we should not all have to pay higher insurance premiums and taxes because some customers use the health care system for nonhealth purposes. As to the definition of medical care—payable by third parties—we have been facing it for many years in the area of plastic surgery. What is reconstructive surgery? What is necessary for the restoration of full function after accidents or to correct deformities so severe as to constitute a severe social or economic handicap or a likely mental health problem? What are mainly aesthetic concerns? The latter are not medical problems and by no means should be covered by insurance. No one has any "right" to avoid the wrinkles of age or the adiposity of overeating or to acquire the beauty not given genetically.

Cosmetic surgery is not covered by most insurance policies, but the taxpayer subsidizes it through subsidies for medical education, health care facility construction, and for most of the activities and facilities involved in health care. Most health care costs are joint costs, unallocable or unallocated by very specific services. It is the jointness of supply, the commonality of suppliers, not third-party payments exclusively, that converts a wider concept of disease into higher costs for us all.

Issues other than cost are related to the proper boundaries of health care. What should be the training of health care personnel, what capabilities should health care institutions encompass in their facilities as well as in their staffing?

Broadly speaking, illness encompasses pathology or a significant departure from the long-term stable condition of an individual; and dysfunction or a disturbance of long-term functioning by an individual. The two overlap and sometimes are interchangeable, but it may be useful to distinguish between a broken leg and influenza. Both are defined with reference to individual norms, not social norms. Since individuals are considered to be very similar to one another as biological organisms, such individual norms tend to be absolute, not relative. A broken leg is dysfunctional for any individual; influenza is pathological. There are of course troublesome cases: the typhoid carrier, for example, for whom the microorganisms are not pathological because in that one respect this individual differs greatly from most others.

There is another concept of illness, one that has vastly enhanced the scope of health care, the empire of physicians. This is a social concept, which is necessarily relative, since social norms may not be rooted in biology in the same way as individual health norms are. Conditions or functioning disapproved on the basis of group or societal norms may be regarded as illness. Much genetic *ab*normality may be classified here. Social disease at one time referred to syphilis and gonorrhea; now we redefine bad or disapproved behavior as sick.

The Medicalization of Life Problems

There is a tendency for all conditions labeled disease to fall within the turf of the medical profession and health care institutions. As a result of antibiotics and other new treatments and preventives, the need for health care should have declined, and health care costs should have dropped as a share of gross national product. Instead we have experienced a vast expansion in medical care costs, facilities, personnel; their appropriation of an increasing share of society's resources (more than doubled in thirty years, and rising). This counterintuitive rise is caused in part by the redefinition of an ever wider range of conditions as disease. We are becoming, by definition, a sick society.

Much of the increased share of resources absorbed by the health care industry represents not higher unit costs but a wider range of services, reflecting better access among the low-income population, new technology, and a wider scope of health services. Improved access for those who need medical care is not to be denied and is a self-limiting cause of rising medical costs. Technology and a wider scope for health services are self-reinforcing rather than self-limiting, and reinforce each other. Health care personnel conceive of new uses for their services, and help generate a demand for them. To curtail health care costs, one must stop the proliferation of disease by redefinition and limit the scope of disease insofar as health care subsidies and insurance reimbursement are concerned.

As we broaden the definition of illness to include excesses (or shortfalls) of drinking, eating, work, or whatever; as we define illness to incorporate deficits of will or character and atypical preferences and behavior, we establish new (and often different) needs for medical personnel and facilities at the same time that we reduce established needs through the progress of public health and medical science. We approach the World Health Organization's (WHO's) unattainable definition: "Health is a state of complete physical, mental, and social well-being and not merely the absence of disease or infirmity."

Extremely small stature, whether genetic in origin or not, need not be regarded as pathological or dysfunctional from an individual standpoint, but may be so regarded by the group. In societies where height is highly regarded, where it offers an important reproductive or survival advantage, its lack is a handicap. Giantism or dwarfism by their definition must refer to a group norm. In the past, people were tall or short according to their genes, or their stars. Now, some who regard themselves as too tall take themselves to a surgeon, who chops off a few inches of their leg bones. Some too short may, if treated at the right time with pituitary growth hormone, gain quite a few inches. Sales of genetically engineered growth hormone exceed any reasonable need; many parents want their children to be six-footers, feeling that such height gives them an advantage in life. Dr. Gavriel Ilizarov in the former USSR cuts leg bone but not the marrow, stretches the cut bone about one twenty-fifth of an inch a day until the desired length is achieved. Now his procedure is also used in the West to make dwarfs taller.[2] Fat can be sliced away with a scalpel, skin made taut, even hair implanted on a bald pate. Much plastic surgery—face-lifts, nose bobs, breast enlargements—corrects no pathology or dysfunction but simply allows the individual to approximate a social norm or, in some cases, ideal. Technology is pitted against nature. Is this medicine, "correcting" departures from some norm or ideal?

Obesity, in the vast majority of cases attributable to overeating, is no longer a state but a disease. Obesity was not formerly considered to be illness; in many less fortunate countries, the expression "My, you're fat!" is considered a compliment. When food was not assured for many, the plumper figure was to be preferred. When a thin body raised suspicions of consumption or tuberculosis, it was feared. Somewhat pudgy women were considered much more attractive than the skinny beauties admired in the United States. They probably were considered more attractive even in the United States a century or two ago, but certainly in Europe. We need only examine the female nudes painted by Goya in the early nineteenth or by Renoir and Degas at the turn of the twentieth century. The skinny silhouettes painted in earlier centuries were spiritual figures and martyrs, admired for their fortitude and faith, not for their shape. Venus de Milo would have weighed at least 160 pounds. The importance of being skinny has never been as great for men as for women, one reason why few men experience anorexia, engaging instead in overexercise, muscle building, and steroids. The overuse of steroids for nonmedical purposes has been recognized as a problem for years.

But why, once food was no longer a problem and tuberculosis until very recently was almost forgotten, should there be a shift in ideal female form toward the emaciated anorexic? We cannot blame doctors for the shift, only for promoting ideal weights that are too low. The health care industry has defined ideal weight in such a way that a large proportion of the population is considered to be obese. A consensus conference held at the NIH in 1985 concluded that 26 percent of the population was medically obese and required medical treatment.[3] Or alternatively, anyone more than 20 percent above the ideal weight for the height was medically obese: a social and not an individual disease. Even this was an upward revision of ideal weight; according to the 1959 Metropolitan Life charts, 70 percent of middle-aged men were obese.[4] Not pleasingly plump, but unhealthily overweight. More recently, one-third of the population has grown into this category, and former Surgeon General Koop, famous for his antismoking campaign, has declared war. Thus a new disease is born. The "cure" for obesity is eating less. But not any longer. Weight control has become a medical specialty. Wards in some hospitals are devoted to reducing weight; a variety of pills (some such as fenfluramine with dangerous side effects),[5] special diets, weight-losing programs, and diet clinics have been developed by the health care industry, to be administered under its supervision.

A lack of exercise is a second reason for obesity, but the solution is no longer simply to exercise. There are medical specialists in this area, who give sometimes conflicting prescriptions, which have changed over time (jogging is out, walking is in). The choice of diets is wide enough to confuse. Some of the clinics and camps specializing in weight loss include exercise under medical supervision as well as technically correct diets, and other clinics concentrate on exercise alone. The exercise fads that have swept the nation, aerobics in particular, have also come under medical supervision in many cases. One does not exercise just for fun anymore, in outdoor activities, in organized sports, if not in the course of one's work. Exercise is part of a medical prescription for health and longevity. At this point, very little of it is covered by insurance, adding to the costs of those who choose not to participate. But we can foresee a gradual expansion of physical therapy, covered by insurance, to include much of the exercise industry. Perhaps the most regrettable aspect of this colonization is that it has qualified the joys of a sedentary life and the pleasures of gluttony without credible evidence that either in moderation is much of a threat to health or life. But, then, the purpose of medicalizing fat and sinew was not health but job creation.

The problem of drug abuse has become a major concern. The approach in the past has been largely on the supply side, beyond the reach of medicine. Our experience with Prohibition should have told us that it does not work very well. Now drug use becomes drug addition, and a new specialty is born, new medical services are stressed to reduce drug use from the demand side. The potential is huge. Fifty-seven million people smoke cigarettes daily; 106 million adults drink an alcoholic beverage at least once a month; and nearly the entire population drinks caffeinated beverages.[6] All three are considered addictive. And then there are cocaine, heroin, their derivatives, and many other drugs thought to be harmful and addictive.

Drinking to excess is a disease. Almost everything done beyond socially accepted norms becomes a disease. "Don't work too hard" is a common greeting that at least retains the idea that it is a matter of individual choice. But the workaholic is a sick person, by the very choice of terms. Persistence becomes clinical obsession. Eating, drinking, working, smoking, almost any habit that meets disapproval becomes the object of clinical attention, therefore by implication a disease, subject to treatment by withdrawal, or habit de-formation techniques, or drugs, spawning new "medical" specialties. No longer bad, but sick. Is drug addiction an illness? Sometimes. But in whose jurisdiction? Medical or psychotherapeutic? There is much battling over turf, which can be found also in treatments for obesity, alcoholism, and many other new "illnesses."

Then there is the subject of abortion. I do not wish to become involved in the perpetual disagreements on abortion rights, only on insurance coverage or its definition as a disease. Pregnancy is not a disease. Abortions in most cases have nothing to do with health care; they are the result of carelessness or change of mind for which the rest of us should not pay. There is a strong case for abortion in the case of pregnant women who have no prospect of providing adequately for a child; but if the woman cannot pay, the responsibility should fall on the welfare system and general taxation, not on the health care system and health insurance premiums. Medicaid finances abortions. Even if financed by taxation and debt, they probably raise prices and insurance premiums slightly for the rest of us because of Medicaid's low reimbursement rates, which induce providers to compensate via higher prices for others. The same is true of pregnancies that are likely or certain to result in highly defective offspring. For the state to assume responsibility to abort raises grave moral issues that should be the responsibility of the parents. The same issue arises with respect to services of medical personnel and facilities to induce pregnancy or to eliminate the risk of pregnancy. We are not talking about illness, but about complying with the wishes of potential parents. Let them pay.

We already have to deal with the moral issue of prolonging or ending the life of the terminally ill or those whose survival means little more than a vegetative existence. Is this health care?

Most of these areas of recent medical invasion, newly defined illnesses, have one thing in common: they represent behavioral choices of individuals. They are diseases that the victims bring on themselves in most, if not all, cases. Do they still have the right to treatment? That is, do the rest of us have an obligation to pay for their treatment? Daniel Callahan says no.[7] They differ from the issue of smoking and lung cancer and other behavioral diseases in that the behavior is a predisposing condition, an intervening variable toward serious medical consequences, not itself formerly regarded as an illness. We propose to treat the predisposing condition, obesity, as a disease. (We do this already for high cholesterol and blood pressure, but these conditions are not usually the result of controllable individual behavior.) Its potential consequences are part of the established medical agenda. (The excuse that obesity and most behavioral conditions are in our genes I consider later.)

Genetic Medicine

Two growth areas that offer almost unlimited scope for expanding the boundaries of medicine are genetic medicine and mental illness. The latter is considered in Chapter 7; here we examine genetic medicine.

We are on the verge of a technological revolution, such as we have not had since the development of penicillin, if not since Pasteur's discovery of the germ theory of disease. Gene after gene has been identified—more than 600 to date—that is associated with higher-than-average risk of incurring particular ailments.[8] DNA tests are available for more than thirty inherited diseases, and this is just a beginning. This revolution will come in three stages. The first, identification of the genes, is upon us. The second, gene therapy, or preventive gene therapy, which will treat or prevent the occurrence of the disease in an individual, is in the early stages of research. The third, much farther down the road, is the prospect of altering genetic inheritance so that offspring will not carry the defective gene. This revolution offers opportunities to prevent illness and to heal, but it also offers almost unlimited opportunities for excess services and services that have nothing to do with health care.

The payoff from DNA identification is not limited to genetic screening. It is helpful in diagnosis, identifying the microorganism that is causing infection. It has led to the ability to manipulate genes to produce better drugs. Insertion of the appropriate human genetic component in rodents permits its replication on a mass scale. Human insulin, the first genetic drug, was created in 1983. Human growth hormone, new vaccines, drugs, and blood-clotting agents followed. It is possible to supplement the body's defenses by replicating the appropriate human cells in large numbers outside the body, then injecting them to fight infection, perhaps someday soon, to fight cancer.[9] It is not this development that raises concern.

DNA identification offers the prospect of enormous increases in health care costs by screening large numbers or the entire population for a rapidly growing number of defective genes. For what genes should screening be conducted? Who should be screened? Screening cannot be conducted for every gene to be identified that may lead to undesirable consequences, nor can everyone be screened for everything. We will have to choose. The first question is the seriousness of the condition for which a genetic propensity has been established. The second question is the probability that possession of a particular gene will lead to a particular illness, a probability in excess of that of those without the gene. Does the defective gene guarantee that the individual who has it will develop the disease or does it just increase the chances slightly? The third question is, what can be done about the illness? Is there a preventive? Is there a cure?

In rare cases, such as Parkinson's disease, those with a single genetic defect will almost certainly develop the illness, and there is neither preventive nor cure. Advance knowledge helps in making decisions on procreation and on dealing with a premature death or disability. Testing to determine genetic propensity for illnesses for which there is no treatment is not health care. There may be a right to know, and the individual who someday will be afflicted may want to know sooner and take appropriate steps. Or he may prefer not to know. But there is no social obligation to bear the costs. In this case, gene analysis is not medical care in any sense.

In other cases, as in breast cancer, those with the predisposing genes are much more likely than the average to develop breast cancer, and to develop it early, but they are not certain to do so. There are treatments, often cures. These are more likely to be effective the earlier the cancer is detected. Such individuals should get mammograms early and often. They need to know this. But perhaps only 5 percent of the population have the predisposing genetic defects. Should all women be tested, or only those with a family history of breast cancer? Most breast cancers occur in women without the predisposing genes, although their risk is much lower. We can already identify individuals almost certain to develop breast cancer before menopause.[10] Once cancer-prone women are identified, then mammograms can be limited to them until, say, age fifty. But what is the difference in outcome between annual mammograms and biennial, triennial? How much difference will this make? Our current knowledge refers to all women in clinical tests and recommends against annual tests; but we need to find out if there is a difference between them and those with a genetic predisposition.

On the other hand, a much smaller proportion of the population have the gene for cystic fibrosis or Parkinson's disease; the rest of the population does not suffer from these ailments. Hence high-risk groups should be tested, but others should not. The problem lies in identifying high-risk groups.

As the number of predisposing genes multiplies, the possibility arises of millions demanding gene analysis for a large number of possible illnesses or disabilities. The additional cost would be in the tens of billions, possibly hundreds, should all demands be met. Who should get gene tests, and when additional tests such as mammograms permit detection of a disease early enough for effective treatment, how often should these additional tests be given and to how many? Some diseases, such as cancers, have numerous predisposing genes, and it may be a long time before genetic analysis can come up with a probability for individuals with a particular predisposing gene or genes. "Yet public demand is likely to lead to widespread testing long before all the glitches have been ironed out."[11] As in breast cancer, once the predisposing gene(s) has (have) been identified for other cancers, there will be frequent diagnostic tests, which will also run well into the billions.

Genetic testing is a Pandora's box, which opens up another Pandora's box. What happens when most of the U.S. population discovers that it possesses genes predisposing toward this or that cancer, or mental ailment, or heart attacks, or the early onset Alzheimer's? Americans do not accept determinism, do not readily submit to fate. There will be an insatiable demand for preventive measures, which will focus on gene therapy, on the insertion of good genes to replace bad genes. It will be a long time before much can be done along these lines; initial experimental efforts have had only temporary effects, but they will be in demand nevertheless.

The advent of genetic medicine also opens wide the floodgates for diagnosis of inherited conditions that are not health problems, and whose treatment is not medical care. Only if one's genetic makeup indicates a high probability of incurring some serious illness or disability can genetic testing be regarded as a preventive health measure; even then, only if there are effective means of coping with the likely disease or disability. If there are no medical countermeasures, then it is an ethical issue, not a health issue.

This revolution will take time. In the great majority of cases there is no single genetic defect whose presence is associated with a high probability of occurrence of a particular illness. More than a hundred genes have been identified so far that appear to be associated with different kinds of cancer. Most illnesses involve several genes. It will take much study to sort out the influence of different genes and be able to predict the effect of a particular combination of predisposing genes.

The third stage, altering the germ cells to eradicate a defect, not only from the individual treated but from any progeny, is now only in the mind's eye of ambitious genetic researchers. There are many who hope it goes no further. Their concern is not cost, however large it might be, but the enormous ethical problems involved should we acquire the capability to tinker with the human race itself. All of us have some bad genes. Learning about them will cause us problems enough, as the knowledge may influence individual choice of mate and decisions on progeny and attitudes toward life in general. Unfortunately, anything that can be done probably will be done.

Why the Excessive Services?

The share of gross national product devoted to medical care should have declined as a result of the antibiotic revolution.[12] It should also have declined because as incomes rise, spending on health care increases less than proportionately.[13] This did not happen because of a flood of costly halfway technologies that at best provided half-cures. A decline in health care spending was precluded by third-party payments and the ability of supply to create demand.

The main cause is the large increase in the ratio of M.D.s to population, resulting in growing surpluses in some specialties, which has contributed to oversupply of services and higher prices. Overbuilding of hospital beds and excess supply of expensive instrumentation such as MRIs have also contributed to oversupply of services and higher prices. Supply largely determines demand; there is abundant evidence that the quantity of services in a medical market is quite sensitive to increases in the number of providers: more tests, more surgical procedures, more visits. Rapid increases in fees, when accompanied by rapid increases in M.D. earnings, cannot be explained in terms of rising costs. If they are not explained by greed, or as the economists put it, the effort to maximize income, how can they be explained? Medical imperialism, the expansion into new areas of testing and treatment, wider concepts of disease, and increasing specialization and subspecialization go hand in hand. They are expressions of oversupply, physicians and hospitals seeking more work.

The claim that specialists in excess supply induce additional demand to render services and perform procedures not medically needed is most strongly supported by the fact that areas with higher M.D. to population ratios not only have higher quantities of medical services per capita but also higher prices. In a competitive industry, larger quantities could be sold only by lowering prices; not in medical care. Additional demand must be induced. It is difficult to maintain that, especially in surgery, areas with lower ratios have fewer operations per capita because they do not have enough surgeons. But the question of how much is enough is not easily answered; physicians disagree.

The statement that a surplus of M.D.s "induces" additional demand is unquestionably correct, but subject to misinterpretation. All physicians induce demand; I know of no one who on his or her own initiative shows up at a doctor's office and demands the removal of a gallbladder or a coronary bypass. That is the job of diagnosis, to determine what if any additional medical tests or services seem required by the symptoms reported or observed. Not all demand inducement is bad.

There are many motives driving physicians and medical establishments to increase their supply of services. Perhaps most important is what economists call income maximization, but others know as greed. Older physicians often express the belief that M.D.s turned out in the past decade or two are much more likely to be motivated by greed than were their seniors. This is an opinion, not established by statistically sound procedures, and even if it were, it would remain opinion. It may be less characteristic of general practitioners than of specialists. Prices are more readily compared for the services of general practitioners. Greed is easier to accept when the doctor is dealing not with a customer but with a liver or vertebra. Dr. Arnold Relman, editor of the *New England Journal of Medicine,* is quoted as follows: "Doctors are more concerned about their economic future than I can ever remember. There is more pressure on the doctor to maintain his income than is good for the public or the profession."

The word "greed" is not used in a derogatory sense but as a simple description. Economic systems are driven by greed and envy; in capitalist systems, greed is the main motor; in socialist, envy. Other motives exist and matter, such as Veblen's instinct of workmanship and a sense of service, or there would be little job satisfaction or quality maintenance. There is no necessary conflict between greed and the highest standards of medical conduct, professionalism, in a technical sense, and the delivery of medical services. But there is a tradeoff in terms of the number of tests, the quantity of services rendered. They may be performed to the best of a good physician's ability, although they should not have been done at all. I could name a prominent neurosurgeon who has a single book in his office, prominently displayed: *Value Line.*

The near-doubling of the ratio of M.D.s to population during the past forty years, from thirteen per 10,000 to twenty-four, is in part justified by the changing age structure of the population, in part by new technologies requiring more doctors. But the increase would have been excessive, the incomes of M.D.s would be down very substantially, many would be unemployed, were it not for third-party payments, which increase demand for their services.

There would be many more M.D.s at lower pay were it not for restricted enrollments in medical schools. One consequence is the establishment of a number of medical schools abroad whose primary function is to train M.D.s for the American market. Another is a flood of immigrant doctors. Of course, lowering average earnings by flooding the market with more doctors does not necessarily lower prices; in general the opposite is true, and raises total costs of medical care by expanding the supply of services rendered.

Once in medical practice, a physician is likely to charge prices comparable to those charged by fellow physicians and to recommend medication and procedures in line with what has become standard practice. It is the thing to do, if he wants to be a member of the club. To charge less may lead to suspicion that his services are of inferior quality. Thus, for most, greed may not be involved; they are only behaving as custom dictates; only a minority charges and recommends what it thinks the market will bear, but this minority in time establishes common standards.

The motive of greed driving the physician to excess testing and treatment can be unconscious in many cases because the same behavior may also be driven by the technological imperative that moves doctors to try new and more tests and treatments, counting no costs. On the other hand, the process of weighing the costs and benefits to the customer conflicts with the technological imperative.

Much is made of defensive medicine as a cause of overtesting and overtreatment, in legitimate self-defense. Liability insurance is estimated to cost $45 million a year, all of which is passed on to customers.[14] No one knows how much additional tests and procedures are the result of fear of litigation, but surely more than the cost of insurance. Much of the defensive medicine, and many of the malpractice suits, are nothing but greed masquerading under the pretense of self-insurance or self-defense or patient rights to cure. Malpractice insurance should reduce the "need" for defensive medicine, but it appears to have the opposite result, since premiums may be based on experience with malpractice. Limitations on the size of malpractice awards, penalties for frivolous suits, and no-fault insurance would greatly reduce the practice of defensive medicine, whatever its true motivation, by reducing both need and excuse. Group practice—in hospitals, HMOs—offers a much better opportunity for M.D.s to keep an eye on each other's work than does private practice. It also provides the means of disciplining and denying access to M.D.s who are not up to snuff. Such an alternative to malpractice suits is both more knowledgeable and cheaper, were it adequately employed, which it is not.

The legal profession, despite innumerable good works, some *pro bono publico* (free of charge), on a net basis is a deterrent to economic growth, a deterrence for which it is well compensated. Nowhere is this clearer than in its contribution to reducing the productivity of health care through malpractice litigation.

We think of malpractice insurance and associated costs in terms of doctors and hospitals. But its equivalent occurs in firms supplying medical products, drug firms in particular. Their prices must consider risks and costs of litigation. So must their premarketing testing and evaluation. The price of DPT (diphtheria, pertussis, and tetanus) vaccine for children rose from 11 cents in 1982 to $4.29 a dose in 1985 primarily as a reaction to suits resulting from the fact that one in 310,000 doses results in permanent damage.[15] The alternative, no pertussis protection, would be much more damaging, but there would be no firm to sue. Some manufacturers have discontinued the production of some vaccines and drugs as a response to the costs and fears of litigation. In addition to higher prices, some drugs and treatments are not available in this country, and the potential beneficiary must get them abroad.

Why excessive surgical procedures? The surplus of surgeons is the main but not the only reason. Take, for instance, coronary bypasses. At first there was considerable uncertainty about the results and unduly optimistic expectations. Thus, too many were performed. Understandably, for hindsight proved sharper than foresight. The fact that bypasses were performed not only on those most likely to gain but on many others who were less promising candidates statistically reduced the resulting benefits. At first it was the only procedure in town. But competing procedures, such as balloon angioplasty, were developed. And evidence that drugs in many cases could make both procedures unnecessary accumulated. One would expect that, as knowledge improved, fewer bypasses on marginal candidates would be performed and that the availability of alternatives would further reduce the number of bypasses. Nothing of the sort happened; the number performed kept increasing. At this point none of the previous explanations suffice. The case of caesarian sections is much simpler. There was little uncertainty about which individuals needed it, what were the benefits and risks, but the number performed has exploded nevertheless. The institution of Medicaid, which gave the poor an ability to pay, was a factor.

Then there is the overprescription of drugs. The total sales of many drugs for specific conditions far exceed the needs of individuals suffering from these conditions. Doctors rarely profit from this, except indirectly, by saving office time and by requiring return visits. It is a way to bring a visit to closure, often expected, or even demanded, by the patient. Drugs are a large factor in iatrogenic illness. Looking at the *Physicians' Desk Reference,* one can find drugs with dozens of possible side effects. No one knows who will be affected by any one of them. New side effects will be found with the passage of time, while some effects listed are speculative possibilities that may not be realized. There is a tendency to stress possible contributions and neglect the risks and medical costs. With the present organization of medical care, an individual may be taking drugs prescribed by several physicians, with no one in charge, no one knowing the entire pharmacopeia inflicted on him. Clearly it is the generalist who should be informed, and who should alert the patient and specialists if needed. With many powerful drugs on the market, and with an aging population taking multiple drugs, the neglected specialty of pharmacology needs more attention. When an individual is taking seven or eight different medicines, no one knows how they may interact, what is really going on chemically.

There are other motives for excessive services and procedures. One of them is the ethical desire to do everything possible, no matter how remote the chance that a particular test or procedure will help the patient recover. The American medical ethic, no different from that of any other American occupation, is not "First, do no harm" but "Do something!" This ethical motivation usually is consistent with the wishes of the patient, and thus the oversupply can be described as responding to the customer's demands. The motivations that conquered this continent are not acceptance or compromise or limited expectations.

Quite a few years ago, in a seminar on health economics with a group of physicians, I stated that with insurance coverage, if nothing were done to rein in the system, we would someday be spending 25 percent of the GNP on health care. One of the physicians saw nothing wrong with this. More recently, in a discussion with a very knowledgeable and experienced health care administrator, I raised the issue of excessive costs resulting from too many CT scanners and MRIs in a large metropolitan area. He did not agree with me; if scanners were more closely spaced, it would take less time for an accident victim to get to one, and a life might be saved as a result. There could not be too many scanners. Unfortunately, duplication of services and facilities is not always for the purpose of improving access; it is one way in which hospitals compete. Staff specialists, or specialists the hospital would like to attract, demand the latest and best equipment. If one assumes that the value of a human life is infinite, then what if saving an additional life costs a few hundred million dollars? The same attitude arises in the area of environmental health and accident prevention. In fact, W. Vip Viscusi has estimated that a new regulation would have to cost at least $100 million per life saved before it was likely to be rejected by OMB.[16] There is always something else, something more to be done, to be tried. If we had firehouses and police stations on every block, undoubtedly a few additional lives would be saved, injuries avoided, crimes prevented, criminals caught. But in this area, we have achieved a reasonable compromise between costs and benefits. People resist paying higher property taxes. Not so in health care.

Then there is what Victor Fuchs calls the "technological imperative." Most M.D.s are highly trained technicians who take great pride in their special skills and want to put them to use. They are more interested in the process perhaps than in the product. This was stressed in their apprenticeship as interns and residents. In this country the special skills in which one takes great pride are not the traditional crafts carried on from generation to generation but the newest skills, never before known; the latest, therefore in American mythology, the best. The customer agrees, he or she wants the latest technology available in a technocratic civilization. Both M.D. and customer are ever on the lookout for new technology, the final product of the industry of discovery and invention that is research and development: "the underlying bias of the technological mindset and its activity orientation . . . that newer must be better and that doing more must be better than doing less; hence the possibility of harm is always a second thought. . . ."[17]

Health care has been dominated by the technological imperative—the belief that new drugs, new procedures, new treatment will cure nearly all disease, including the failures of will and character. This belief is most likely to prevail in teaching hospitals, and is independent of method of compensation. It caters to a desire to learn and a desire to play with new technological toys. If a patient were aware of the risks and uncertainties involved in new drugs and new procedures, he or she might opt against them. But, then, the M.D. may not know either.

Notes

1. Rick J. Carlson, *The End of Medicine* (New York: Wiley, 1975).

2. "Perestroika for Bones," *Economist,* June 25, 1988, 87–88.

3. Thomas Moore, *Lifespan—Who Lives Longer and Why* (New York: Simon and Schuster, 1993), 144–46.

4. Gina Kolata, "Obesity Declared a Disease," *Science* 227 (March 1, 1985): 1019–20.

5. Deborah Barnes, "Neurotoxicity Creates Regulatory Dilemma," *Science* 243 (January 6, 1989): 29–30.

6. Murray E. Jarvik, "The Drug Dilemma: Manipulating the Demand," *Science* 250 (October 19, 1990): 387–92.

7. Daniel Callahan, *What Kind of Life—the Limits of Medical Progress* (New York: Simon and Schuster, 1990), 208.

8. Victoria Conti, "New Insights into Cancer, Psoriasis, and Other Major Health Problems," *NCCR Reporter,* March/April 1994, 4–11.

9. Steve Olson, *Biotechnology—an Industry Comes of Age* (Washington, D.C.: National Academy Press, 1986).

10. Yoshio Miki, Jeff Swensen, Donna Shattuck-Eidens, et al., "A Strong Candidate for the Breast and Ovarian Cancer Susceptibility Gene BRCA1," *Science* 266 (October 7, 1994): 66–71; and Richard Wooster et al., "Localization of a Breast Cancer Susceptibility Gene, BRCA2, to Chromosome 13q12-13," *Science* 265 (September 30, 1994): 2088–90.

11. Rachel Nowak, "Genetic Testing Set for Takeoff," *Science* 265 (July 22, 1994): 464–67, esp. 467.

12. Lewis Thomas, "On the Science and Technology of Medicine," in *Doing Better and Feeling Worse—Health in the United States,* ed. John Knowles, 35–46 (New York: Norton, 1977).

13. Victor Fuchs, *The Health Economy* (Cambridge, Mass.: Harvard University Press, 1986), 87, 281.

14. Patricia Danzon, Mark Pauly, and Raynard Kington, "The Effects of Malpractice Litigation on Physicians' Fees and Incomes," *American Economic Review* 80 (May 1990): 122–27.

15. Gina Kolata, "Litigation Causes Huge Price Increases in Childhood Vaccines," *Science* 232 (June 13, 1986): 1339.

16. W. Vip Viscusi, "The Value of Risks to Life and Health," *Journal of Economic Literature* 31 (December 1993): 1912–46, esp. 1943.

17. David Mechanic, *Inescapable Decisions—the Imperatives of Health Reform* (New Brunswick, N.J., and London: Transactions, 1994), xi.

7

Mental Illness

Mental illness is a bottomless pit. It is the one area that medical imperialism has failed to colonize. At this time it would be difficult to claim that there is excessive demand; the opposite claim is more plausible. Demand falls far short of need; whether it falls far short of opportunity to benefit from treatment is another matter. Demand falls short in part because of limited insurance coverage for treatment of mental illness. But the main reason is a large gap between the psychotherapists' broad concepts of what is mental disorder that should be treated and the much more limited public concept of mental disorder. There is also a residual stigma attached to seeking help for mental or emotional disorders. It does not fit in the germ model of disease as an external cause.

A further reason for limited demand is that many needing psychotherapeutic help, even viewed from the individual or family members' perspective, refuse to recognize their need and seek help. For those who do seek professional help, the average number of sessions with a psychotherapist is only 2.5, meaning that the vast majority of those who seek help meet at most twice with professional therapists.[1] Fifty percent do not make it to the first agreed-upon meeting. It would be difficult to argue that this is enough to do what can be done for them. Stephen Kopta and associates examined outpatient treatment for sixty-two symptoms and found that the minimum number of weekly sessions needed is eleven and the average is fifty-eight.[2]

The implicit collusion between excess supply by providers and excess demand by customers characteristic of medical care is absent in the case of mental illness. Hence the need for a separate chapter.

How Much Mental Illness?

Twenty five percent of Americans are estimated to experience depression severe enough to require professional help at some time in their lives.[3] The

National Institute of Mental Health (NIMH) concludes that 20 percent of the population will have a diagnosable mental disorder at some time in their lives.[4] About 6 percent of the population can expect to experience clinical depression within a six-month period. Robert Michels and Peter Barzuk estimate lifetime prevalence of mental disorders as 33 percent of the population, 22 percent if we exclude substance abuse.[5] A recent survey by the Institute for Social Research of the University of Michigan found that 48 percent of the population experience some mental disorder during their lives (25 percent experiencing an affective disorder, primarily major depressive episodes).[6] Fifty percent of all office visits are reported to be prompted by mental or emotional problems, with no diagnosable physical causes.[7] How this figure was arrived at, how physicians could know categorically that there were no physical causes, particularly with their bias toward physiological causation, or how the absence of detectable physical symptoms is evidence of emotional or mental disorder, I have no idea. The point is that M.D.s, not just psychiatrists, believe that mental and emotional disorders are extremely widespread. None of these estimates includes the next big mental disorder: substance abuse of nicotine, which has just been added to the psychotherapeutic repertoire. Yet only 1 percent of the people think that mental illness is a major health problem, and 55 percent do not believe that it exists.[8]

Extending Coverage to Mental Illness

If mental illness were fully covered by insurance, and in particular if the definition of mental illness were the psychotherapists' and not the public's, there is little doubt that the increase in demand would be huge. Would the demand for mental health care be excessive? That is not a simple question. It depends partly on what can be accomplished via psychotherapy. Insurance coverage, apart from its effect on costs to the customer, would help legitimize consumer use of psychotherapeutic services. The demand for mental health care is more sensitive to cost than other health care. A study by Thomas McGuire of imposing full coverage for mental health on small firms in Connecticut suggests that demand will increase two and a half times.[9]

How would full coverage for psychotherapy affect total costs for medical care? Kaiser Permanente in California and the San Joaquin Foundation for Medical Care found that providing coverage for psychotherapy greatly reduced the use of medical, surgical, and health services. Kennecott Copper also found that coverage reduced total medical costs and that it reduced absenteeism.[10] These experiments were conducted in the 1960s and 1970s.

Substantial progress has been made in the treatment of schizophrenia and depression since then, and there has been some reduction in the stigma associated with receiving psychotherapy. The chemical model of mental illness, which has gained much ground since with the development of numerous drugs, helps relieve the individual of guilt or responsibility for his condition, increasing the likelihood of seeking help. The coverage in these studies did not include some of the newly invented or discovered "disorders," which if covered would unquestionably greatly increase total medical costs. HMOs are in a better position to trade off physical and mental treatment (often joint ailments) than the fee-for-service market. Willard Manning and associates estimated that providing ambulatory mental health services free would increase demand 133 percent above demand with 95 percent co-payment, but found little support for an offsetting effect on physical health care or total medical costs.[11] Since less than 5 percent of the population eligible for free care received any care, there could not have been a sizable effect. They did find that the average user had eleven visits per year; this is over four times the national average, which includes people with and without insurance coverage for mental illness. Thus the impact on total medical costs remains an open question, but I suspect that, as most of the population eventually accepts the concepts of mental illness or disorder rife among professionals, medical costs would rise, and coverage could make the increase quite large. It is estimated that only one out of five people who need psychotherapeutic help ever seek it. One problem with determining the size of the potential market and therefore the extent of coverage and potential costs is that the experts who make recommendations are professionals with some vested interest in expanding their markets. Depression alone is estimated to cost $45 billion a year, but much of that is loss of work, not treatment cost.

The Providers

Who are the providers? They are a mixed bag in training qualifications, perceptions, practices, and therapeutic orientation. There are very few common standards. "Responsible reviewers have guessed that there may be 100 or 140 schools of psychotherapy—all of them in the mainstream."[12] Drop a zero, and that is still confusing. Success depends more on the abilities of the therapist than on the methods used. The concept of mental illness is not one on which all suppliers agree. Psychiatrists, with their conventional medical training, are prone to define as illness any problems with which they deal. They are likely to disagree often with other mental health practitioners on concepts, causes, and certainly on appropriate treatment.

The psychiatrist has a bias toward chemical therapy, whereas other practitioners, with different training and perspective, have a bias toward understanding the role of the individual and the family situation. Clinical psychologists, psychiatric social workers, and once most important and still of some consequence, religious and community leaders and family members, see many of the same problems not as illness or even individual disorder but either as an individual's inability to cope with personal problems—family difficulties, interpersonal relations, frustrations resulting from school, job or career conflicts or failures, death of loved ones—or as personal idiosyncrasies, atypical personality or behavior. These differences in concept in turn lead to different therapist behavior. If depression is not the problem but only a side effect of the problem, Prozac could not even be coping with symptoms but with the symptoms of symptoms.

There is no consensus on what is mental illness, and who is mentally ill, on what therapy should be followed, or even on what constitutes a "cure." Some mental illness is predominantly biochemical, and often long-term drug therapy is the only available treatment. But for many more sufferers, although they may benefit in the short run from drug therapy, long-term improvement if not "cure" depends on a deeper understanding of their problems, on changing behavior or even possibly personality.

It is strange that when there was no medical treatment for mental illness, psychologists could not be reimbursed by insurance companies; they had to work under the supervision of a psychiatrist. Now that numerous drugs are useful in treating some mental disorders, psychologists have obtained autonomy in most states. The battle over turf remains and will continue as long as there is so little certainty about origins, contributing circumstances, diagnoses, and appropriate therapies. In many cases, there should be a division of labor and collaboration between medical and psychological approaches and corresponding therapists. But the division of labor is breaking down, as psychologists in state after state obtain the right to prescribe as well as hospital staff privileges. The same growth of specialization observed in medicine is also occurring among psychologists. It is a phenomenon associated with rapid growth in the number of doctors of psychology. The clinical psychologist, originally the equivalent of a general practitioner, may now specialize in children or the elderly or substance abuse or sleep disorders.

Treatment

Until recently there were no medical treatments for mental illness. Schizophrenia, which accounts for 40 percent of long-term hospital beds, remains largely resistant to efforts to cure. Chlorpromazine, introduced in 1952, and succeeding drugs with less dangerous side effects can moderate episodes and help prevent further episodes, but it is not clear that they do more than treat symptoms, and there are reservations about the damage they can cause. Choice of drugs is an unresolved issue, as is dosage; side effects are troublesome.[13]

Drugs for depression and mania are also of fairly recent origin. Lithium was introduced in this country in 1970. Chemical treatment for depression is more successful than for schizophrenia.[14] But even now, prescription of antidepressants may represent a temporary cure and a longer-term preventive for those serious depressions and manic-depressive conditions that are of chemical origin, but only a palliative for those—the great majority—that are perhaps normal responses to such unfortunate circumstances as the loss of loved ones or loss of a job, responses that are self-correcting in time. They are like prescribing decongestants for a common cold, for which there is no cure. But acute depressions, untreated, often lead to suicide, forcing therapists to take preventive action.

For depression not attributable to problems of living, for manic-depressive psychosis, and for schizophrenia, our understanding is quite limited, and our treatments of uncertain effectiveness. Bad psychotherapy can be worse than no psychotherapy. The magnitude of the problem as seen by psychotherapists does not measure the need for treatment; it suggests the need for research, which is badly underfunded relative to research on other major health problems.

We are sure that there is a genetic basis for some schizophrenias, perhaps excess dopamine receptors, but also that it takes environmental conditions—stress perhaps—to trigger the onset of the illness, and to trigger additional episodes.[15] Manic depression and some major depressions also have a genetic basis, expressed in chemical imbalances or a deficiency of serotonin, but most do not. Thirty to 40 percent of those believed to have a manic-depressive gene never develop the illness.[16] The evidence of a genetic predisposition for schizophrenia includes family histories and the high probability that if one identical twin has it, the other will also develop it.[17] But replication of genetic studies for both illnesses has failed; it appears that not a single gene but different genes are implicated.[18] The assertion that the proportion of the population exhibiting schizophrenic behavior is roughly the same in different ethnic groups as evidence of its genetic basis[19] is puzzling; neither genetics nor environment would lead us to expect this. (Besides, the incidence of the major mental illnesses seems to be particularly high among the Irish.[20]) It is equivalent to asserting that blond hair cannot have a genetic basis, since its incidence varies widely.

Of course, every effort is being made to find a mutant gene for every disorder, to identify some difference between brain chemicals or structure in those who suffer from them and those who do not. This is in keeping with the germ model of disease; a single cause, in this case not external to the individual but physiological, not psychological. Life is not that simple. For one thing, correlation is not causation. Identification of a chemical overabundance or underabundance, too many dopamine receptors, or not enough serotonin in major depression does not provide a cause for schizophrenia, nor does it prove that schizophrenia from other causes brings about the abnormal concentration of the brain chemical. Also, there is no sharp differentiation between schizophrenics and others in terms of abnormal concentrations: some schizophrenics do not have them, some who show no symptoms do. Here we have a statistical relation, not an individual diagnostic one. "No functional or structural changes in the brain can unequivocally be associated with the disease [schizophrenia]."[21] It appears that not a single gene but several, either severally or in combination, predispose toward schizophrenia and toward manic depression.

Some mental illness is traceable to viruses. Borna virus—a virus found in horses and sheep in Germany and Switzerland—antibodies were found in Philadelphia mental patients but not in the control group.[22] Other mental illnesses are attributable to diet; in Guam, for instance, from eating false sago seed (and kuru in New Guinea).[23] But these environmental explanations are limited in scope.

Neurotoxic chemicals in the environment may account for some mental disability or illness. Lead is the best known. But the search for harmful chemicals has concentrated on carcinogens. We know that some psychoactive drugs cause temporary and perhaps lasting disturbance in emotional balance and mental functions. Some of these are illegal drugs; others are psychiatric medications.

Another environmental explanation, this one sociological, is applicable to most mental illness. It has been noted in this country and others that the incidence of mental illness is inversely related to socioeconomic status. At first glance this suggests environmental causation. But causation can run both ways: poor people are subject to much more stress than the well-to-do and not surprisingly suffer more from a variety of mental disorders. Or individuals who suffer from serious mental disorders experience income and career deprivation, moving down to lower socioeconomic status even if initially they were well off. There is evidence of income loss to the mentally ill, which is particularly large for schizophrenics. Bruce Dohrenwend and associates have investigated the alternative explanations in Israel.[24] Schizophrenia occurs more than four times as frequently among high school dropouts than college graduates; substance-abuse disorders twenty times as often; and major depression less than twice as often. Dohrenwend and his associates concluded that the higher incidence of schizophrenia among low-income groups is mainly attributable to the adverse effects on income; poverty is more an effect than a cause. On the other hand, low socioeconomic status and associated higher stress is the major contributing factor to depression among women, and antisocial personality and substance abuse among men; low status is largely a cause.

These are not either-or alternatives, in theory or in behavior. Long-term changes in biochemical mechanisms can result from behavioral states. There is interaction. In some schizophrenics and depressed patients, certain psychological states may lead to changes in neuroregulator activities.[25] And environments, too, are inherited.

Predisposing environment cannot be defined just in terms of socioeconomic status; stress and frustration are found in every class, so it is not surprising that so are schizophrenia, depression, and other mental illnesses. We can safely predict that the huge increase of out-of-wedlock births, single-parent families, and divorces will raise the incidence of "mental" illness for a long time to come.

The vast majority of mental disorders, as defined by the professionals, at this point appear to be behavioral-environmental in origin. This is not to say that some individuals are not genetically more prone than others to such disorders (e.g., alcoholism), but genetic propensity is not genetic determinism. The relevance of this belief is that neither reducing the incidence of mental illness nor curing it can be left to medical professionals. It is largely a social and a cultural problem.

Why, then, should mental illness have been the concern of physicians specializing in psychiatry, when in most cases their medical training was irrelevant, and the appropriate treatment could be best provided by psychologists and counselors, priests, parents? This is another example of medical imperialism, the medicalization of emotional disturbances and aberrant behavior. Medicalization may eventually be justified in part, as we improve drug therapy for schizophrenia and establish the genetic basis for some mental illness and find ways to correct it. But a good share of what passes for mental illness treated by psychiatrists should remain the proper domain of counselors, social workers, and psychologists, not medical psychotherapists with a certain bias toward labeling disturbed states as illness and toward chemical salvation. Much of it should not be regarded as illness at all, but as an understandable response to life circumstances that may or may not be the most appropriate one.[26]

It is not psychiatrists alone who practice imperialism in this field. Psychologists are just as guilty. Part of the problem is that anything psychiatrists feel competent to deal with is automatically an illness; that is what physicians are trained to treat. Psychologists expand their territory not by labeling everything as illness, but by stressing, first, their training to help deal with emotional disorders and to some extent, less so than social workers, with the consequences of social disorganization, and, second, their skill in attempting to change interpersonal relations, not simply the outlook and behavior of a single individual. These issues are not exclusively professional or medical. Insightful relatives, friends, schoolteachers, community leaders, and religious leaders may be able to do well, with the advantage of established personal rapport with the "patient." Of course, when they do well, the disturbed individual is unlikely to seek professional help.

What Is Mental Illness?

We discussed treatment before considering what mental illness is, because that is the way mental illness has been managed; some drugs work sometimes, sometimes not, we know not why. Some psychotherapeutic techniques work for some, not for others. Working means inducing acceptable behavior, but what is acceptable changes over time and varies across class, race, ethnic group, country.

What is madness? The imagination of poets, the dreams of saints, the creative vision of inventors and discoverers, the literal and exclusive pursuit of self-regarding gains? Or a state of mind, elation and depression, or megalomania, schizophrenia? Mental states that were formerly regarded as normal individual variations or temporary responses to circumstances or were universally admired have been reclassified as illness, to be treated and if possible "cured." Yet attitudes once regarded as reprehensible, cardinal sins such as pride, greed, and egoism, are preached as the normal attributes of individualism. The shamans, seers, oracles of old civilizations became the witches of the Middle Ages, who in turn became the schizophrenics of our time.

What is acceptable behavior? What is illness? Is individual idiosyncrasy amusing, annoying? What aberrant behavior is regarded as mental disturbance, what criminal, what sinful? Kleptomania or theft? Pyromania or arson? Temporary insanity or murder? If mental disturbance, how does one deal with it? Directly by professional psychotherapist or intermediated by family, community, alternative therapies? What is the attitude of the disturbed individual and mediating agents toward psychotherapy?

Behavior that is clearly harmful to the individual experiencing it or to individuals subjected to it may be deplored and may call for intervention. But what kind of intervention? Police? Parson? Or psychotherapist?

There is the physiochemical model of mental illness toward which medicine aspires. And then there is the psychological model, favored by psychologists and social workers, which in turn can be partitioned into the sociological (interaction between the individual, family members, and other individuals important to him) and the sociocultural, characteristic of an entire society or class or ethnic group. None is complete, nor are they mutually exclusive. The choice of models influences attitudes toward the objectionable behavior and the choice of therapies.

The diversity among practitioners makes it difficult to agree on the nature of mental illness or disorder and what should be done. These issues refer to origins or causes of mental illness. But what behavior constitutes mental illness? Long after we may have settled the question of sources or causes, there will be disagreement about unacceptable behavior and about the locus of responsibility for change: again, parent, police, parson, psychotherapist.

A lack of consensus between the different kinds of practitioners is to be expected. But one finds it even among respected psychiatrists. The extreme view espoused by psychiatrists R.D. Laing, Thomas Szasz, and Peter Breggin, among others, is that either there is almost no mental illness or what we call mental illness is only a rational response to an individual's experience and circumstances.

Laing says that except for chronic schizophrenics, he has difficulty discovering signs of psychosis in persons he is interviewing.[27] He views the behavior of a schizophrenic not as symptomatic of a disease but as the expression of his existence, his effort to cope with insecurity. Leifer attacks the medical model of mental "illness": "Medicine and psychiatry differ in every important respect except the rhetoric used to describe them."[28]

Szasz states: "Mental illness is a myth. Psychiatrists are not concerned with mental illnesses and their treatments. In actual practice they deal with personal, social and ethical problems of living . . . psychiatrists cannot be expected to solve ethical problems by medical methods." [29] He also objects to the label of mental illness because it undermines personal responsibility by assigning blame for antisocial behavior to an external source, whether chemical imbalance or childhood mistreatment. Szasz opposes accounting for normal behavior in terms of motivation but abnormal behavior in terms of external causes over which the individual has no control.[30]

Breggin's work is a detailed, documented challenge to the use of antipsychotic drugs.[31] He feels that depression should not be treated with drugs because it is a psychological, not a physiochemical, disorder. He warns against mood-altering drugs, Prozac in particular, claiming that its dangerous side effects have been understated or overlooked, that its effectiveness is limited, and that it can cause the very condition it is intended to treat. And it diverts the provider from tackling the real problems, which he regards as psychological, not chemical. Needless to say, psychiatric organizations, most psychiatrists, and the drug manufacturers disagree. Two-thirds of mental patients are treated with major tranquilizers. They produce indifference, apathy, reduced spontaneity, and docility, and a permanent disfiguring neurological disease, tardive dyskinesia. They permanently damage higher centers of the brain, producing irreversible psychoses, generalized brain dysfunction, and other effects similar to those of lobotomy.[32]

Electroconvulsive shock produces numerous small hemorrhages in the brain and cell death; that is how it achieves its results, which are a serious loss of memory and mental abilities. The damage is the cure.[33] As to antidepressants, some include or turn into neuroleptics in the body; tricyclic drugs can also produce tardive dyskinesia and tardive dementia, mental dysfunction, and memory impairment.

Two conclusions impressed me. First, drug effects are independent of biological or psychological disorder; they are the same for schizophrenics, manic depressives, compulsives, bulimics, victims of other anxiety disorders, *and* "normal" people. (Prozac helps prevent severe anxiety attacks of patients with panic disorder or obsessive-compulsive disorder; it is prescribed also for sensitivity to criticism, fear of rejection, lack of self-esteem, and deficiency in ability to experience pleasure.)[34] Second, the same drugs used to treat a variety of mental illnesses were first used to control prisoners and rebellious children and were used by the KGB to torture and subdue political dissidents.[35] Their main effect is to control and subdue, one reason they are used by veterinarians.

Most providers who prefer psychotherapy to drugs still would claim that in some cases short-term drug treatment is necessary before the patient can be treated psychotherapeutically, although I doubt Breggin would concede this. Psychotherapy does not always succeed; when it does not, is the drug treatment (or electroconvulsive therapy) always worse than the disease?

The new drugs emptied the mental hospitals. But many who left ended up swelling the homeless population. Before reading Breggin, I believed that their problem was a failure to continue taking medication, the lack of a follow-up system to assure that they did. This is undoubtedly the case for most. But now I wonder if, for some, the problem is having taken too much medication for too long.

Before dismissing this dissident minority of psychiatrists, recall that Egas Moniz, who developed the surgical lobotomy, sometimes performed with icepicks thrust into the cortex through each eye socket, a procedure now thoroughly discredited, won a Nobel prize for it in 1949. Keep in mind also the strong bias of medically trained psychiatrists toward chemical salvation, a bias widely shared by the general population.

My purpose is not to propound a particular view, although I lean toward the psychosocial interpretation for ideological if no other reason. The point is that there is no agreement on what qualifies as mental illness, what brings it about, what conditions qualify, what is the appropriate "treatment," or even what constitutes a "cure." Surveys carried out to establish which therapeutic approach is best to my mind border on the absurd. Best for which client? Which therapist? When mutually inconsistent approaches turn out to be about equally effective, one wonders about their validity. Better forget about comparing approaches until we know more about what is being approached.

Psychotherapeutic Imperialism

The opposite of Laing's view, that we are all mentally ill to some degree some of the time, is not as modern as one might think. Benjamin Rush, physician to some of the Founding Fathers and a signer of the Declaration of Independence, is also considered the father of American psychotherapy. He believed that liars were mentally ill, which makes all of us sick.[36] The belief that human beings are not morally responsible has been developing for two centuries. Karl Menninger, leading psychiatrist in the mid-twentieth century and president of the American Psychiatric Association, saw crime as a medical (psychiatric) problem.[37] This perspective, carried to its extreme, implies that we need, not prisons or churches, but mental hospitals. No cardinal sin escapes the clutches of psychotherapy, and few cardinal virtues. Recently this view has been reinforced by progress in identifying genes associated with particular illnesses.

The writings of opponents of the medical model of mental illness appear to have been in vain, largely because of the development of the pharmaceutical treatments Breggin condemns. Perhaps, however, they contributed to a new terminology: mental disorder. The concept of mental illness has undergone a vast expansion in recent decades. The percentage of the population believed to need treatment has grown accordingly. Now alcoholism is the second most prevalent mental illness, although in the near future smokers may join the list and outnumber alcoholics. In 1993 the American Psychiatric Association voted to classify a severe form of premenstrual syndrome (PMS) as a depressive disorder, believing it occurs in only 3 to 5 percent of women. The National Organization for Women (NOW) opposed the idea, considering the definition overly broad and applicable to 40 percent of all women.[38]

Leading professional psychotherapeutic associations conclude that women suffering from severe postmenstrual tension require their professional services; so do the 20 percent of the population classified as obese (one-third are now considered overweight). Fifty million Americans may require treatment for depression. Much habitual behavior becomes an addiction over which individuals have little or no control (it is in their genes), but nevertheless it is a mental illness requiring psychotherapy and/or drugs. Many but not all alcoholics apparently have a genetic predisposition, yet not all with such a predisposition end up alcoholics. The current word is that 65 million smokers are addicts requiring treatment as clients, although the appropriate gene has not yet been identified. Compulsive shoppers may be next on the agenda.

The latest manual of mental disorders lists nicotine-related disorders, including nicotine dependence and caffeine-related disorders (anxiety and sleep disorders), but not caffeine dependence.[39] The manual has a code for Trichotillomania, or recurrent pulling out one's hair resulting in noticeable hair loss (is baldness a disorder now?), for sleepwalking disorder, and for frotteurism, or sexual urges or behaviors involving touching or rubbing against a nonconsenting person. Among personality disorders are histrionic personality disorder (some ethnic groups watch out!) and narcissistic personality disorder, which should become epidemic if attempts to induce it (it's now called "self-esteem") in schoolchildren succeed. Codes that transgress the territory of other agents of society include identity problem, which refers to uncertainty about issues such as long-term goals, career choice, friendship patterns, sexual orientation and behavior, moral values, and group loyalties; religious or spiritual problem, such as loss or questioning of faith, conversion to a new faith, questioning of spiritual values; phase-of-life problem, associated with entering school, leaving parental control, starting a new career, and marriage, divorce, and retirement; and adult antisocial behavior, which includes the behavior of professional thieves, racketeers, or dealers in illegal substances.[40] A truly global empire!

Is drug addiction a medical problem? Sometimes, but I must confess great skepticism. There is physiological addiction (e.g., to heroin) but not as much as some claim. But no one becomes physiologically addicted after a single experience with cocaine or heroin, much less cigarettes. It takes weeks, months, or years. Crack is highly addictive, but psychologically more than physiologically. Many millions have given up smoking in the past two decades. I suspect that most addiction is purely psychological. That there are differences between those who take up smoking and those who do not, those who quit and those who do not, is well established.[41] There are addictive personalities. I once knew a man who was hooked on peanut butter; he would sit down with a jar and a spoon, and could not stop until he had cleaned out the whole jar. I know a man addicted to swimming;

if he misses his dip more than one day, he is ready to climb up a wall. These are behavioral traits, not diseases, for which only the individual should be responsible. Drug addiction is a self-inflicted behavioral obsession; why should others pay? What about obesity? Most obese people eat too much and exercise too little. Overeating, overdrinking, or using drugs has much less to do with genetic propensities than with what used to be called character or self-discipline. To give in to "irresistible" impulses is now a mental disorder, a scientific version of demonic possession, as Szasz called it.

In 1890 there were perhaps as many drug users relative to the population as there are today; earlier users were addicted to cocaine cola and cocaine-laced cough syrup advertised in the Sears, Roebuck catalog. But no one was robbed for drug money, no one was murdered. One wonders whether the current problem of addiction to illegal drugs would be regarded as an illness, or a mental illness, if no crimes were committed other than the sale and use of illegal drugs. The criminal by-product is a public safety problem, not a health problem.

Some advocate the legalization of drugs. Drugs would become very cheap, sold through supermarkets and drugstores below prices that suppliers could possibly charge and still profit. (The result would be a body blow to several nations to our south and the elimination of any surviving "fashion" in drugs.) Solutions always create their own problems. Users will commit fewer crimes. But what will the hundreds of thousands making a living by importing, transporting, and selling drugs do once this source of income is gone? Will crime go down, or up?

This imperialism of professional associations together with the search for biological excuses fits well with the twentieth-century theology of victimization as it has evolved in the United States. The therapist is out to prove that we are all victims (of our genes, if nothing else). In the end, so are the culprits, whether their behavior is bigotry or harassment or a major criminal offense. The view that there is no crime, only illness, appears to be gaining ground. Note what has been happening to convictions of the perpetrators of major crimes, to sentences, and to effective punishment. Here we go beyond genetic determinism; they were sexually abused or otherwise mistreated as young children, and forever after they must commit crimes for which they are blameless. This "tyranny of the past" is an endless regression, passed on from generation to generation even in the absence of genetic inheritance.

I do not question that these are real problems for the individuals involved and that many of them could benefit from help. But medical? Psychiatry is time-consuming; there are few shortcuts or opportunities for delegation to less skilled technicians, one reason for reliance on pharmaceuticals, which are great time-savers.

The supplier is willing to deal with a vast array of problems and issues. Can he be equally competent in all? The vast scope calls for a specialization that in fact is occurring, or for all-purpose drugs. Is the alleged short supply attributable in part to the propensity of psychiatrists to venture beyond their proper field? The new agenda of psychotherapy is in contention with physicians other than psychotherapists, not just with psychologists, who may try to treat obesity or alcoholism, as they already treat depression, some of whom may develop a specialty in dieting, alcohol, or drug withdrawal. The only constraint is on the side of demand, not supply. The size of the medical market for mental health will ultimately be set by customers, not practitioners.

If most of the people who need psychotherapy do not seek it, and many if not most of these who seek it drop out prematurely, why are the providers so hell-bent on expanding the scope of mental "disorders"? Is there really a shortage? Only 20 percent of those who need help are seen by psychotherapists, although many others consult primary-care physicians and other counsel. If all those who needed care sought it, practitioners would be in very short supply; it would be some years before their numbers could expand to meet needs. It may be this combination of competition for turf with others and the reluctance of victims to seek help that requires the creation of so many mental disorders, some of them bordering on the ridiculous, such as "restless legs sleep disorder."[42]

Behavioral Correctness

With whose "incorrect" behavior should the public and the health care establishment be concerned? First, with those whose behavior poses a threat to others, for example, dangerous lunatics and uncontrollable psychopaths; second, with those unable to cope with their environment, who become burdens, wards to others; third, those who suffer unduly. Finally, what about those whose performance is far below their potential because of psychological problems—unhappiness, frustration, indolence, sociopathy, or what have you? Here we must step carefully. Most people's performance is far below their potential, assuming we can measure that, and for many it is by unconstrained choice—they have goals other than the performance principle, the work ethic. Are they to be labeled mentally ill because they prefer leisure, choose not to plan ahead, or refuse to respond to challenges? Because they are narcissistic or histrionic? Because they are looking out for themselves singlemindedly or have difficulty adjusting to divorce or retirement? Few psychotherapists would label all these conditions mental illness, even if their association lists them as mental disorders. They are trespassing on territory not their own. It is not clear to me that it is their business to set societal norms or attempt to enforce them. Persons performing acts of great benevolence at great personal sacrifice, or heroism at great personal risk, are never declared mentally ill and prescribed Prozac (except rarely by would-be heirs who fear a fortune slipping from their future). They are considered responsible for their own behavior. Why not many of those of whose behavior we may not approve?

One reads about Soviet dissidents consigned to mental hospitals and subjected to appalling treatments and dismiss it as another extreme instance of political disregard for the rights of individuals. And it was just that. But it was also something else: an extreme case of defining and diagnosing deviance as a disease. Printing, distributing, even reading underground newspapers became a symptom of mental illness, greatly widening the scope for the practice of "psychotherapy." A family member, trade union, business organization, or polyclinic doctor could have the dissident committed.

The use of drugs to achieve some social norm or social ideal of personality, mood, and behavior that happens to be that of an extroverted, forever-smiling simpleton could empty our graduate schools and riddle the ranks of executives, political leaders, and inventors. Compulsive, driven behavior is almost a requirement for them. The entire populace would be reduced to a field of placid cows that moo sweetly in the meadows—this in a society that allegedly values pluralism, diversity, individuality.

I grew up in another country, another culture. My childhood photo album is filled with grim, unsmiling faces—like Grant Wood's "American Gothic." It was past the time when heads were held in vises to hold them steady during long exposures. Perhaps they had bad teeth. But no, life was hard, adults were sober and serious, and children aped their seniors. Later photos, taken in this country, had everyone showing their teeth. If extroversion drugs lead every stranger, every telesalesman to address me by my first name (too many do already) and intrude a feigned intimacy, give me Grant Wood!

The Demand for Psychotherapy

This vastly expanded scope for psychotherapy, although widely shared among the psychotherapeutic professions and accepted by some avant-garde liberal groups, has not yet been adopted by most of the population. The supplier is willing, but the market demand is not there. Still, it may be only a matter of time. More extensive coverage of psychotherapy by insurance would contribute toward legitimizing it in the eyes of a skeptical public.

The willingness to seek help depends crucially on individual self-perception. One reason for the fading of the stigma once attached to mental illness and professional help is the weakening of the view of the individual as independent, self-reliant, in control of his or her own life. The same reasoning applied to the family viewing itself as self-sufficient, in command of its affairs. The breakdown of the extended family, even of the nuclear, paternalistic family, plus the weakening of religious and other community ties, have reduced mediating alternatives.

Not too long ago, psychotherapy was something the customer and the family regarded as shameful, to be kept secret; seeking help was an ego-deflating admission of failure. Seeking professional help was a tactic of desperation rarely resorted to. This attitude has changed dramatically, although not among all ethnic groups. Now, being in therapy is fashionable; therapy has become a fad among some groups that can afford it. There are high-fashion therapists, whose prestige is maintained by the fact that, unlike high-fashion couture, their services cannot be expanded indefinitely. For those who see a therapist regularly for ten or fifteen years, there is no therapy, perhaps no fashion. Just another addiction.

It is easier to accept chemical treatment for physiological illness manifested as manic depression or schizophrenia or a variety of mood disorders than psychotherapy for a psychological illness. And it is easier as well as cheaper to swallow legal happiness pills, Prozac, than to rely on psychotherapy. Perhaps the experience of the drug culture, which used LSD and other drugs to create illusions, "abnormal" behavior, contributed.

With the decline of rugged individualism, there is a desperate search for biological determinism on the side of the customer as well as the psychiatrist, ridding the victim of any responsibility. Whatever I do, whatever I am, it is all preordained. If not in my genes, then in my childhood experiences; my parents are to blame in either case, for the genes I inherited or for their behavior toward me. I am a victim of the tyranny of the past.

In America and other advanced societies there is a different current that is even more demeaning of the individual. It views the mentally ill, not as victims of a disease that should be treated, but as mere symptoms of a "sick society." Treatment may be counterindicated because it would "sicken" the individual, that is, bring him to terms with a sick society. The proper agenda then becomes revolution or a redesign of society. This view carries the medical model far beyond the aegis of M.D.s or psychotherapists, making every dissident a doctor. That is not quite the intention of some psychologists and psychiatrists who propounded the vision of a sick society (incidentally conceding that they could not treat or cure their patients), but it is the consequence. Health becomes a function of the environment, not just the physical environment with its overload of pollutants, but of the total environment: psychological, social, political, economic.

While the Calvinist doctrine that ye shall know a man by his works has been largely discarded, the expectations that went with it have, if anything, been inflated. The individual is indoctrinated from an early age that unlimited possibilities are open; he is infused with great expectations that, however reasonable they may be for a few (e.g., growing up to be president), are impossible for the vast majority. Preserving self-esteem without attainments or accomplishments is an impossible task. Thus disappointment, frustration, ego threat are inevitable outcomes. Some accept, some are unhappy, others exhibit behavior variously labeled neurotic or psychotic.

In a society that claims to believe in meritocracy, and to a considerable extent practices it, self-esteem is fragile and always at risk, for it is derived from individual accomplishment, not from membership in a family, class, region, or ethnic group, in which therefore individual accomplishment reflects only on the self and knows no boundaries. It is a society where upward (and downward) mobility is widespread, and seen to be open to most.

Consider anorexia nervosa, a disease of the ego, a perversion of the American achievement syndrome, an involution of individualism, widespread in achievement-motivated subcultures of North America, almost unknown in cultures where the ego is subordinated to some collective id. It is called an eating disorder because it takes the dramatic form of extreme emaciation. The individual, most often a female, feeling inadequate and helpless, shrinks the limits of her world to the environment she can control, practicing tyranny over her own body, in the unshakable belief that she is fat. The same phenomenon, in the Middle Ages, was a qualification for sainthood.[43]

Among males, not culturally predisposed to think that thin is beautiful, compulsive exercise and body building are the common forms of ego disease involving tyranny over one's body, although they are rarely recognized as another manifestation of the same sickness. Both are negative responses to feelings of inadequacy, withdrawals into a lonely megalomania over a personal world radically simplified to a single simple goal.

Willingness to seek professional help seems to vary inversely with the strength of family and community relations. The close-knit family first assumes responsibility and then relies on community services and facilities: alternative therapies, religious and social support. Only as a last resort does it turn to professional psychotherapeutic services. One would expect Afro-Americans to be at the forefront in seeking help because the breakdown of the family is more advanced in this community than elsewhere. The reverse is the case, primarily because the providers are regarded as alien institutions that do not understand them or have rapport with them. With Hispanics, language is a greater barrier. Members of both groups tend to rely on alternative therapies first, with conventional psychotherapy as a last resort.

In time, any stigma attached to psychotherapy should diminish, in every ethnic group, and disappear in some. But the current evidence is that, even among those who do seek psychotherapeutic assistance, only 50 percent return for the first agreed-upon therapy interview, and 70 percent discontinue treatment before the fifth session.[44] Phillips was of the opinion that most people seeking psychotherapeutic help only need that opening interview, but that is an overoptimistic belief. There is still a widespread reluctance to seek help, and to continue treatment. This high rate of attrition has hampered efforts to study outcomes.

Changing Concepts of Mental Illness

In previous ages, individuals hearing voices, speaking in tongues, or exhibiting behavior we might now label schizophrenia might have been oracles, seers, shamans, holy ones; later, as recently as the eighteenth century, they were evil witches and warlocks. The concept of insanity or highly deviant behavior as an illness is fairly recent. Phillipe Pinel (1755–1825) pioneered the concept of insanity as an illness and unchained his insane prisoners. In England the idea was invented as a means of sparing "witches" from burning at the stake. Insane asylums at first were not places for treatment but for quarantining those judged insane; the emptying of leprosaria provided the buildings. With the fading of belief in demonic possession, people found it difficult to explain deviant behavior except as the responsibility of the deviant; it could be labeled sin or, in some cases, crime. In the popular mind, this is still largely true. But the attribution of deviant behavior to mental illness goes back at least two centuries, to Benjamin Rush.

The Catholic church and several Protestant denominations still believe in demonic possession, which, though extremely rare, is distinguishable from schizophrenia. Rites of exorcism have a long history. Thirty-four percent of the people in the United States believe that the devil is a personal being who directs evil forces and influences people to do wrong, according to a 1981 Gallup poll.[45] Psychiatry calls possession something else, finds it all too common, assumes that much of it is inborn, biological and not theological, and performs its own rites of exorcism.

Ethnic and Religious Differences

Social groups tend to differ in what they regard as unacceptable behavior and in what they label as mental illness, and in their willingness to seek psychotherapy. "That which is regarded as 'illness' in one society may be regarded as merely one aspect of the normal and healthy life in another." [46] They also differ in the types of mental illness commonly found. Schizophrenia and those depressions believed to have a strong genetic component are said to be found with much the same frequency everywhere; why is not clear. But attitudes toward them vary. Other illnesses vary widely in frequency because of differences in environment, as well as in concepts of unacceptable deviant behavior.

Diagnosis is often difficult. Patients with "problems in living" considered psychotic by the majority of Americans are not so considered in the United Kingdom. Americans diagnose schizophrenia too freely; many so diagnosed would be diagnosed by the British as neurotic or suffering from personality disorder. [47]

More pertinent are the differences in acceptable behavior found among ethnic groups within the United States. Most Mexican Americans do not regard hearing voices as evidence of mental illness; nearly all anglos do. [48] Puerto Ricans and Cubans accept hysterical outbursts resembling epileptic seizures as normal. [49] Obsessive-compulsive behavior is accepted, even demanded, toward desired goals, by some Asian ethnic groups. Suspicions rejecting all evidence, sprouting conspiracy theories like weeds after a summer rain, characterize ethnic groups from what I call "bazaar societies" along the Mediterranean and the Middle East, in which all unfavorable developments outside one's control that are not attributable to natural causes are viewed as conspiracies, in which the schizoid tribal morality—one code for "we," another for "they"—is the norm. One might be tempted to call such societies paranoid, and they are by comparison with Western societies, but the attributes are cultural and only incidentally individual.

On the other hand, one might with equal plausibility label at least the upper echelons of society in America as hopelessly neurotic, driven to overachievement by the meritocratic ideal, with equality of opportunity making the ego threat of failure pandemic. Consider the numberless casualties of the civil war between the desires and limitations of the self and the internalized expectations and demands of family and society: the victims of anorexia nervosa, the thirty- and forty-year-olds floundering through life "trying to find themselves."

Shall we treat neurosis on a case-by-case basis, accept it and ignore it in most cases, or turn off the engine of growth and progress that generates a pandemic of neuroses as its exhaust product? There are large costs in either case: a complacent, static society, on the one hand, a dynamic society on the psychotherapeutic couch on the other. There is a third alternative: a shift from conformity toward tolerance. How much, what range of diversity is acceptable? Tolerance moderates the tradeoff between mental health and economic growth. Acceptance of a diversity of styles gives individuals a choice, so there is no stigma in not being driven. The expression I have heard from Asian immigrants, "What are your credentials?" has been displaced by the new narcissistic slogan, "How do you feel?"

Jews are the group most open to psychotherapy, whose concepts of mental illness are closest to those of psychotherapists. Whereas almost 50 percent of Jewish respondents suggested psychotherapy as the best resource for a family problem, only 24 percent of Catholics and 31 percent of Protestants agreed. Jews will resort to psychotherapy for relatively trivial problems, such as a child's academic performance or decision to leave home. Asian Americans are among those least prone to seek help, and those who do are likely to have serious problems, with a high rate of psychosis.[50] Many ethnic groups—Puerto Ricans, Greeks, Chinese, Norwegians—deal with their reluctance to cope with mental illness by regarding it as physical ailment and seek medical rather than psychotherapeutic help. They differ in their concepts of causes; the Irish, for instance, are likely to blame themselves; the Greeks and Puerto Ricans, someone else.

In terms of demands from psychotherapy, there are large differences. Most ethnic groups demand prompt results, will not put up with extended treatment, and care little for understanding. (They almost compel psychotherapists to use drugs.) Jews again are at the other extreme; they are suspicious of a direct problem-solving approach, wanting to gain understanding of the nature of the problem first. They hesitate to rely on drugs, fearing their long-term effects. They are generally prepared to undergo lengthy insight therapy. WASPs also value insight therapy.

Among the less-educated Hispanic and Afro-American population, practices intended to drive out evil spirits and restore afflicted individuals to health or good fortune are widespread. Unlike possession and exorcism in established religions, these practices derive largely from African and Indo-American beliefs and practices, with a veneer of Christian motifs. And possession is common, not rare. These practices are resorted to before considering conventional psychotherapy. How much they reduce the demand for psychotherapy is unknown. They must have a substantial effect, or people would cease going to the faith healers, *santeros, curanderos, spiritistas,* witch doctors.

In Santeria, as practiced among Cubans, but also among other Hispanic people, the *santeros* are likely to send the sick to physicians and mental health facilities for diagnosis and treatment. *Santeros* believe that they help in this regard and that their ability to appease or deter evil spirits is complementary to the work of conventional therapists. "It is not surprising that the authoritarian counselling given by power-manipulator santeros and reinforced by supernatural consent and coercion seems to be effective among many people who have been reared in an authoritarian family structure." [51] The Puerto Rican *botanica,* or folk pharmacy, adds spiritism (the teachings of Allan Kardec) to the practices of santeria. The faithful consult the medium for all problems, including exorcism of evil spirits.[52]

Afro-American folk healers believe that all illness is theoretically preventable. They stress causes, not symptoms. Natural illness is caused by the environment or reflects Divine punishment. Unnatural or magical illness may be caused by worry or by evil influences or by sorcery. The healer may come by his powers by birth or learning or have them conferred during an altered state of consciousness.[53] Because Afro-Americans tend to mistrust all institutions except their own churches, it is likely that the availability of folk healers significantly reduces the use of conventional mental health facilities.

The various healers have in common that they do not separate physical and mental illness, science and religion, and that most of them deal with common problems of money, jobs, love, together with illness, whereas the psychotherapist is not concerned with the whole range of human afflictions and only the psychiatric social worker may try to deal with most of them explicitly. Altered states of consciousness, which might be labeled psychotic by the standard psychotherapist, are a characteristic of many folk healers and are part of their process of dealing with problems presented to them.

What we foresee is a convergence of much of the population on the prevailing professional attitude. Psychotherapy becomes perfectly acceptable, even fashionable, among some; it replaces intermediary structures of family and community, displaces alternative therapies, all of which play a diminishing role. We can foresee reduced acceptance of aberrant behavior and its classification as mental illness; rejection of individual (and family) responsibility for behavior; and the dominance of the philosophy of victimization, externalization of causation, which becomes attributable to another generation, another class, another race, or, for those who can do none of these, to abstract nouns such as society and business, of which we form no part.

Insurance coverage will greatly expand the demand for mental health care. But enlargement of the popular concept of treatable mental disorder to converge on that of psychotherapists could bring about a larger increase.

Notes

1. E. Lakin Phillips, *Patient Compliance—New Light on Health Delivery Systems in Medicine and Psychotherapy* (Lewiston, N.Y.: Hans Huber, 1988), 58–59.

2. Stephen Kopta, Kenneth Howard, Jenny Lowry, et al., "Patterns of Symptomatic Recovery in Psychotherapy," *Journal of Consulting and Clinical Psychology* 62 (October 1994): 1009–16.

3. Gina Bari Kolata, "Clinical Trial of Psychotherapies Is Under Way," *Science* 212 (April 24, 1981): 432–33.

4. Constance Holden, "Giving Mental Illness Its Research Due," *Science* 232 (May 30, 1986): 1084–85.

5. Robert Michels and Peter Marzuk, "Progress in Psychiatry" (first of two parts), *New England Journal of Medicine* 329 (August 19, 1993): 552–59.

6. Ronald Kessler, Katherine McGonagle, et al., "Lifetime and 12-Month Prevalence of DSM-III-R Psychiatric Disorders in the United States," *Archives of General Psychiatry* 51 (January 1994): 8–19.

7. A.M. Kleinman, L. Eisenberg, and B. Good, "Culture, Illness, and Care: Clinical Lessons from Anthropologic and Cross-Cultural Research," *Annals of Internal Medicine* 88 (1978): 251–58.

8. Holden, "Giving Mental Illness Its Research Due," 1084.

9. Thomas McGuire, "Estimating the Cost of a Mental Health Benefit," in *Economics of Mental Health*, ed. Richard Frank and Willard Manning, 242–62 (Baltimore: Johns Hopkins University Press, 1992).

10. Constance Holden, "Psychology: Clinicians Seek Professional Autonomy," *Science* 181 (September 21, 1973): 1147–50, esp. 1147. See also Mark Dodosh, "Psychiatrists Fight against Further Inroads by Psychologists in Mental-Health Market," *Wall Street Journal*, August 20, 1981, 29.

11. Willard Manning, Jr., Kenneth Wells, Naihua Duan, et al., "How Cost Sharing Affects the Use of Ambulatory Mental Health Services," *Journal of the American Medical Association* 256 (October 10, 1986): 1930–34.

12. Eliot Marshall, "Psychotherapy Works, but for Whom?" *Science* 207 (February 1, 1980): 506–8.

13. Michels and Marzuk, "Progress in Psychiatry." See also W.T. Carpenter and R.W. Buchanan, "Medical Progress, Schizophrenia," *New England Journal of Medicine* 330 (March 10, 1994): 681–90; Gary Taubes, "Will New Dopamine Receptors Offer a Key to Schizophrenia?" *Science* 265 (August 19, 1994): 1034–35.

14. Constance Holden, "Depression: The News Isn't Depressing," *Science* 254 (December 6, 1991): 1450–52. See also Constance Holden, "Depression Research Advances, Treatment Lags," *Science* 233 (August 15, 1986): 723–26.

15. Deborah Barnes, "Biological Issues in Schizophrenia," *Science* 235 (January 23, 1987): 430–433.

16. Gina Kolata, "Manic-Depression Gene Tied to Chromosome 11," *Science* 235 (March 6, 1987): 1139–40.

17. Robert Plomin, Michael Owen, and Peter McGuffin, "The Genetic Basis of Complex Human Behavior," *Science* 264 (June 17, 1994): 1733–39, esp. 1734–35.

18. Deborah Barnes, "Troubles Encountered in Gene Linkage Land," *Science* 243 (January 20, 1989): 313–14; Robin Sherrington, Jon Brynjolfsson, Hannes Petersson, et al., "Localization of a Susceptibility Locus for Schizophrenia on Chromosome 5," *Nature* 336 (November 10, 1988): 164–67; Sevilla Detera-Wadleigh, Lynn Goldin, Robin Sherrington, et al., "Exclusion of Linkage to 5q11-13 in Families with Schizophrenia and Other Psychiatric Disorders," *Nature* 340 (August 3, 1989): 391–93; Miranda Robertson, "False Start on Manic Depression," *Nature* 342 (November 16, 1989): 222.

19. Jane M. Murphy, "Psychiatric Labeling in Cross-Cultural Perspective," *Science* 196 (March 12, 1976): 1019–28, esp. 1027.

20. See Monica McGoldrick, "The Irish," in *Ethnicity and Family Therapy*, ed. Monica McGoldrick, John Pearce, and Joseph Giordano, 310–39 (New York: Guilford Press, 1982).

21. Deborah Barnes, "Biological Issues in Schizophrenia," *Science* 235 (January 27, 1987): 430.

22. C.R. Rott and S. Herzog, "Detection of Serum Antibodies to Borna Disease Virus in Patients with Psychiatric Disorders," *Science* 228 (November 15, 1985): 755–56.

23. Roger Lewin, "Environmental Hypothesis for Brain Diseases Strengthened by New Data," *Science* 237 (July 31, 1987): 483–84. See also Peter Spencer, Peter Nunn, Jaques Hugon, et al., "Guam Amyotrophic Lateral Sclerosis—Parkinsonism—Dementia Linked to a Plant Excitant Neurotoxin," *Science* 237 (July 30, 1987): 517–22.

24. Bruce Dohrenwend, Itzhak Levav, Patrick Shrout, et al., "Socioeconomic Status and Psychiatric Disorders—the Causation-Selection Issue," *Science* 255 (February 21, 1992): 946–52.

25. Jack Barchas, Huda Akil, Glenn Elliot, et al., "Behavioral Neurochemistry: Neuroregulators and Behavioral States," *Science* 200 (May 26, 1978): 964–73.

26. George Engel, "The Need for a New Medical Model: A Challenge for Biomedicine," *Science* 196 (April 8, 1977): 129–36.

27. R.D. Laing, *The Divided Self* (New York: Random House, 1960), 28. See also R.D. Laing and A. Esterson, *Sanity, Madness and the Family,* 2nd ed. (New York: Basic Books, 1971).

28. Ronald Leifer, *In the Name of Mental Health—the Social Functions of Psychiatry* (New York: Science House, 1969), 25.

29. Thomas Szasz, *The Myth of Mental Illness* (New York: Harper & Row, 1961), 296, 298.

30. Thomas Szasz, *Insanity—the Idea and Its Consequences* (New York: Wiley, 1987), 346, 352.

31. Peter Breggin, *Psychiatric Drugs: Hazards to the Brain* (New York: Springer, 1983), 23–28.

32. Ibid., 23–25.

33. Ibid., 25–28.

34. Peter Breggin, *Toxic Psychiatry* (New York: St. Martin's Press, 1991).

35. Ibid., 21–25.

36. Szasz, *Insanity,* 188.

37. Ibid., 57.

38. "Severe PMS called 'Depressive Disorder,' " *Washington Post,* May 29, 1993, A17.

39. But see Eric Strain, Geoffrey Mumford, Kenneth Silverman, and Roland Griffiths, "Caffeine Dependency Syndrome—Evidence from Case Histories and Experimental Evaluations," *Journal of the American Medical Association* 272 (October 5, 1994): 1043–48.

40. *Diagnostic Criteria from DSM-IV*™ (Washington, D.C.: American Psychiatric Association, 1994).

41. Isaac Lipkus, John Barefoot, Redford Williams, and Ilene Siegler, "Personality Measures as Predictors of Smoking Initiation and Cessation in the UNC Alumni Heart Study," *Health Psychology* 13, no. 3 (May 1994): 148–55.

42. Stuart A. Kirk, "A Last Dance with Freud," *Newsweek,* October 13, 1986, 15. A different perspective is offered by Robert Yoakum, "Night Walkers," *Modern Maturity,* September–October 1994, 55, 82–84.

43. Rudolph M. Bell, *Holy Anorexia* (Chicago: University of Chicago Press, 1985).

44. Phillips, *Patient Compliance,* 58–59.

45. Szasz, *Insanity,* 286.

46. Anthony F.C. Wallace, *Culture and Personality,* 2nd ed. (New York: Random House, 1970). ch. 6, 209–44.

47. John Townsend, "Labeling Theory," *Science* 196 (April 29, 1977): 480, 482.

48. Amado Padilla and Rene Ruiz, *Latino Mental Health: A Review of the Literature* (Rockville, Md.: National Institute of Mental Health, 1973), 19.

49. Nydia Garcia-Preto, "Puerto Rican Families," in *Ethnicity and Family Therapy,* ed. Monica McGoldrick, John Pearce, and Joseph Giordano, 164–86, esp. 174 (New York: Guilford Press, 1982).

50. Monica McGoldrick, John Pearce, and Joseph Giordano, eds., *Ethnicity and Family Therapy* (New York: Guilford Press, 1982), 384, 221, 11, 174.

51. Mercedes Sandoval, "Santeria as a Mental Health Care System: An Historic Overview," *Social Science and Medicine* 13 (April 1979): 137–51.

52. Mary Ann Borrello and Elizabeth Mathias, "Botanicas: Puerto Rican Folk Pharmacies," *Natural History* 86, no. 7 (August–September 1977): 64–73.

53. Loudell F. Snow, "Sorcerers, Saints, and Charlatans: Black Folk Healers in Urban America," *Culture, Medicine and Psychiatry* 2 (1978): 69–106.

8

The Excessive Demand
for Medical Care

You can't take care of everyone. The demand for
medical care is infinite.
                    —Enoch Powell, U.K. Minister of Health Affairs

Having discussed the amazing ability of physicians to generate additional demand, to the point that even greatly overstaffed specialties have very high average earnings, we now turn to consumer demand for medical care. We seek to understand, first, how consumers can be persuaded to increase their demands at the will of the supplier and, second, how excessive demand is independent of the influence of the health care industry.

It is difficult to distinguish between the excessive demands of consumers for medical services and the ability of an oversupply of M.D.s to generate additional demand for their services.[1] But there are limits to supply-induced demand, and we foresee M.D.s joining lawyers as disaster-mongers. On the one hand, without autonomous excess demand, some of the oversupply cannot occur. On the other hand, without an excess supply, excessive demands cannot be met. They are interdependent. There is some implicit collusion. The decision to see a physician in the first place is entirely up to the consumer. But what happens next is at the suggestion of the M.D. and the discretion of the customer. Better-informed individuals use more medical care. But the effect of their information on number of follow-up visits is negligible.[2]

Demand and Prices

Suppliers and consumers share many of the same attitudes. Neither is constrained by price, only by insurance coverage. Even medical costs, that is, the risks involved in any treatment as distinguished from economic costs, are often slighted if not ignored. Statistical concepts are averaged over large groups, not directly applicable to specific individuals, specific episodes of illness, specific procedures performed by specific M.D.s. Most M.D.s and most consumers are prepared to try procedures of uncertain benefit, of unknown risk.

One reason for demand insensitivity to price (cost) is that the customer rarely knows in advance what services will be needed, at what cost, and how much of the cost will be out-of-pocket cost. That is one reason why, although there are large differences by income, education, ethnicity, and insurance coverage in tendency to see a physician in the first place, these differences tend to disappear with regard to subsequent visits and services.

Chapter 4 considered consumer reactions to lower prices, specifically insurance coverage. In this chapter we do not ask, what about the relationship between demand and price, but, why do consumers demand as much as they do when prices allow them to pay, and even when they do not? Is there a tendency toward excessive demand, which can be freely expressed when costs are covered by insurance? In markets for other goods and services, as long as they cannot be resold, most people limit their purchases of shoes (Imelda Marcos excepted), haircuts, and cars. Is medical care different?

The Right to Health

Milford Rouse, in his inaugural address in 1967 as president of the American Medical Association, said, "We are faced with the new concept of health care as a right rather than a privilege." [3] The idea that we all have a right to unlimited good health has replaced the view that we all have a right to good medical care. [4] Attitudes in the 1970s attempted to repeal the fact that life is unfair, that some fine people are sick and some bastards are healthy, that some have defects, suffer accidents, and experience debilitating disease, while others do not. Hundreds of billions have been spent in a refusal to concede that life is inherently unfair, that destiny does not deal out ability and opportunity to enjoy health, or anything else, equally. The right to health care, if not the right to health, helps explain the growth of health insurance and the demand for universal coverage.

The demand for health services functions at a number of thresholds. First, the threshold for illness: what departure from a state the individual regards as normal warrants concern as a symptom or an illness? Second, how much of a departure from normal warrants recourse to formal health care services? These benchmarks distinguish between perceptible conditions that have and do not have behavioral consequences, and between responses through self-diagnosis and treatment and through recourse to professional care. Once action is taken, what abatement in symptoms is regarded as sufficient to discontinue self-treatment or recourse to professional care? Finally, what are the standards of health professionals for effectiveness that determine what treatments, for what conditions, are in fact available? These standards determine the effective supply of health services. This succession of thresholds and standards is hierarchical. Only on the initiative of customers can professional standards come into play. Somehow all these barriers to professional health care have been lowered. Doctors complain that too many of their visits are from the "worried well." And too many of their services are for newly discovered diseases for which they have no cure, and for conditions only recently defined as illness. The World Health Organization (WHO) definition of health, patently unattainable, has been widely adopted by the public: "a state of complete physical, mental, and social well-being and not merely the absence of disease or infirmity."

Medical care, once considered an investment, has become predominantly consumption; a declining share of that consumption can be reasonably classified as necessity or convenience services, an increasing share can only be labeled luxury by an impartial observer. From the consumer's point of view, the boundary between necessities, conveniences, and luxuries has shifted markedly; some services that once would have been considered luxuries are now regarded as necessities. The results of a Harris poll concluded that most people think that everyone should get the best medical care.[5] The best is a luxury, which by definition cannot be available to all. What is to be done about second-best care if everyone is to get the best?

The more affluent a society, the lower the threshold of discomfort it is willing to tolerate.[6] There has been a breakdown of the ethical distinction between need and desire.[7] Gains are not matched by subjective perceptions of improvement in health. Ours has become a "sick society."

Changing Expectations

Expectations in this culture—perhaps in any culture—tend to outrun attainments, and that is not a bad thing; it helps us to keep moving forward. Our attitudes toward health and illness and disability have changed dramatically. Even a generation or two ago most people accepted some aches and pains, fevers and coughs as normal; arthritis and other common accompaniments of aging were accepted with some grace. Normal blood pressure was 100 plus one's age. Granted, in the past little could be done about lost limbs or crippled joints, for which there are now adequate artifical replacements, and not much about lowering blood pressure. We should not accept disabilities that were formerly irreversible, for which we now have good treatment. But the change in attitude goes beyond recognition of the new art of the possible. The attitude appears to be that the impossible takes a little longer; if we can send men to the moon, why can't we . . .

This has become a hypochondriac society. Now a moderate fever is enough to generate acute anxiety attacks, even a dash to M.D.s or emergency rooms. Many households can display more drugs, vitamins, and dietary additives than the little black bags of M.D.s making house calls only half a century ago. Medical progress has contributed, but so have third-party coverage of medical costs and sick leave. Sick leave (whoever heard of such a thing in the nineteenth century?) was invented recently and has expanded in duration, even as the need for it has been reduced (better health, work that is less physically demanding). Many have come to regard what was once considered malingering as a rightful extension of their annual leave.

What will knowledge of the genetic basis of many diseases do to popular attitudes toward health and sickness? Will it generate a feeling of hopeless determinism, a default of personal responsibility? To the extent that the genetic propensity may eventually be subject to correction, one can anticipate a mass movement in that direction. Priorities will have to be set. There will be excessive demand for genetic testing, for genetic cures, unreasonable demands for research.

Lewis Thomas believes that the biggest source of waste in health care is the public conviction that medicine can accomplish much more than is possible.[8] The combination of excessive expectations and halfway technologies has prevented the cost of health care from falling, as it should have done as a result of the development of antibiotics to fight infections.

The Technological Fix

The demand for the use of new technology, the latest technology, whether called for or not, enabled by third-party reimbursement, constitutes much of the excessive demand. New technology and new knowledge that widen the scope of medical treatment raise the demand. New technology and new knowledge that improve the efficiency or effectiveness of medical treatment reduce the demand for medical care. (Efficiency refers to cost reduction, whereas effectiveness refers to benefit enhancement. In many cases the two go hand in hand.)

Do any new technologies reduce the scope of medical care? No, in the broadest sense of health care over a lifetime; yes, in terms of demand for the services of doctors and nurses and institutional facilities. Some new technologies open up the possibility of self- or home treatment. Yes again, if the new technologies lead to the prevention of illness. Consider the impact of fluorides on the demand for dentists! This new technology can be implemented by dentists, by public health authorities through fluorida- tion of water, or directly by individuals through use of fluoridated tooth- paste. The public has opted mainly for water treatment, which does not involve the medical care industry or individual action. But this is an excep- tion. New technology has been biased toward extending the scope of treat- ment and increasing the effectiveness of existing treatments, not toward cost reduction; hence its net contribution is to increase demand and raise costs.

New demands made feasible by new technology are not per se excessive. But consumer insistence on all possible measures, no matter how low the prospect of payoff, the demand for the latest experimental technology, is part of the problem. This demand is encouraged by publicity, which has oversold medical needs and medical treatments; and by experimental find- ings, which do no more than question existing practices or suggest new research hypotheses through experiments with a few rats and a baboon. These reports are picked up by the press and television and are disseminated to a public that misinterprets (as may the media) their significance. In part, there is the rush to publish results of research, which has to do with tenure, promotion, pay in universities especially, personal advancement in other organizations, and the competitive race to patent.[9]

Although much of the medicalization of the human condition, of life- styles, is the outcome of job- and income-seeking behavior among health care practitioners in the context of a receptive cultural environment, some of it derives from technological breakthroughs. Conditions formerly beyond medical influence, such as epilepsy, or some forms of mental illness, or diabetes, become incorporated within the agenda of medicine. Destiny and fatalism give way to hope and directed effort. Or conditions perfectly under the control of the victim, the result of lifestyles, such as overeating, over- drinking, and a lack of exercise, are exported to the medicinate because the cure—a lifelong reduction in eating, restricted diet, regular exercise, self- denial—is considered far more painful and onerous than the occasional swallowing of pills or even minor surgery. Many believe in chemical salva- tion from all sins. An extreme case is the surgical removal of fat; diet pills are a milder form of the surrender of self-control to a chemical tyranny. Even when there is no medical prescription, there is a demand that one be developed, so we may avoid available treatments or preventives viewed as too high cost in terms of time and self-discipline. We indulge on a large scale in happiness pills, nepenthe pills.

The Sick Society

Finally, there is the growth in the past generation of the "me first" mentality, which demands the best and the latest and counts no cost. The "me" generation, the "I am the world" mentality, is also the mentality of hypochondria. Narcissism may seek self-esteem through athletic prowess, steroids, plastic surgery, anorexia. Face-lifts, breast enhancements, hair transplants, drug treatment used to regulate growth or to improve the performance of athletes, all utilize medical personnel and facilities. Nor are medical contributions to improving performance limited to sports. None are health related, unless one chooses to widen the definition of health to include self-esteem. The supply is willing, but growth depends on demand, which depends on insurance coverage, on who pays. Currently, most of these procedures are not covered by insurance. Some would argue that even without insurance coverage, there is excessive demand, but that is a debate about values, not health.

Illness can be an objective reality, a subjective state, or a societal construct. At the same time that illness as an objective reality has been greatly reduced, it has greatly expanded as a subjective state and a social construct. The sick role is the medicalization of deviance, which frees the individual of responsibility; it is legitimate deviance.[10] It has come to incorporate deviant conditions formerly characterized as sin or crime: compulsive overeating, gambling, theft. "Each civilization defines its own diseases. What is sickness in one might be chromosomal abnormality, crime, holiness or sin in another. Each culture creates its response to disease."[11] The physician exonerates the sick from moral accountability for illness. Americans demand social responsibility for health care, but refuse to admit individual responsibility for their own health.[12]

If one examines trends in per capita days of restricted activity or bed days or days lost from work, one finds a gradual increase for young and old alike in the past twenty years.[13] I cannot believe that sickness as an objective reality is on the rise; as a subjective state, as a social construct, yes.

This narcissistic insistence on rights without responsibility and with no concern for costs imposed on others dooms a system such as the one we now have to absorb indefinitely larger shares of total resources until declines in living standards and the burdens borne by the young and healthy in behalf of the aged and ill become so obvious and so painful that they will spark a revolution discarding the present system despite the vested interests of medical groups, hospitals, insurance companies, and government bureaucracies.

Risk and Uncertainty

Americans are reported to be risk-prone—far more so than most people. They are a nation of immigrants, descended from pioneers, with a very high rate of geographical and job mobility, living in a society that leaves so many choices to the individual, that allows, even encourages, upward and, inferentially, downward mobility. That is the key—downward mobility— that explains why Americans, risk-prone otherwise, should be risk averse in matters of health. There is no chance of an El Dorado, a promotion, a payoff of any kind. Starting with normal health, there is only one way to go, downhill. The American in a normal state of health, which is most of us, is risk averse.[14] He exhibits the "worried well" behavior that adds to medical costs. Risk aversion means that people are willing to pay, via insurance, two to three times the cost of trivial, cheap, and commonplace medical services that should not be covered by insurance at all, since there is little uncertainty about their occurrence and modest cost. On the other hand, those who are seriously ill or impaired are often willing to face great odds and bear much uncertainty for the sake of returning to normal health or competence, again adding to medical costs. Our attitudes toward risk and uncertainty border on the schizophrenic. Thus both the risk aversion of the healthy and the risk-prone attitudes of the sick contribute to higher medical costs.

We wish to be assured that drugs do no harm. This consideration was for a long time the philosophy of the Food and Drug Administration; its unwillingness to accept the findings of tests conducted in other countries, and a tightening of requirements after 1962, lengthened by years the period for testing and for review and final approval of a drug. The ancient Greek prescription "First, do no harm" was supplemented with a requirement that a drug demonstrate effectiveness as well. This contributed to delay, a further increase in costs of FDA approval, and reduced effectiveness by raising drug prices as well as delaying their introduction. The cost of introducing a new drug was greatly increased, first to some $50–60 million and now reported to be over $200 million. One does not need to arrive at a judgment on health consequences to reach a verdict on impact on costs of medical care; they have to go up. The introduction of new drugs, around 350 a year at the time the amendments were passed, dropped sharply to fewer than 100, and is still far short of the previous rate. It is not clear that this represents a loss. But the approval system is too heavily weighted in the direction of safety, which cannot be assured until many years of use, and even then only with an improved system for reporting side effects. It ignores the question, is the new drug sufficiently more effective than existing drugs, or with significantly fewer dangerous or unpleasant side effects, to justify its invariably higher cost? What are we to conclude? Postponing the introduction of drugs, or refusing to introduce or produce them, means that disease goes untreated and victims suffer and sometimes die. "Premature" introduction or the introduction of drugs with limited effectiveness is associated with fail-safe demands of the public, grasping at straws by the sick, and the economic interests of pharmaceutical companies.

The FDA and the legislators who constrained its choices only reflect popular opinion. Consider the numerous legal actions against pharmaceutical companies whose products have met FDA approval. Sometimes many years later, harmful effects are identified; or some highly sensitive individuals will be harmed even if a drug or a vaccine is perfectly safe for the vast majority. These adversary procedures (which often reflect greed rather than fail-safe attitudes, but would not be profitable without such attitudes) raise costs of treatment; they sometimes result in the denial of treatment to many sufferers; and they sometimes result in the cessation of production of, or failure to develop or introduce, drugs and vaccines that might benefit many. Whereas the risk prone drive up demand for medical care, the risk averse also drive up its costs.

In one respect risk aversion, together with excessive expectations, increases medical costs without question, and that is through malpractice litigation, much of which results from the unwillingness of the customer to assume any liability for the inevitable uncertainties associated with treatment. The problem here is not just a fail-safe attitude but one that attributes liability to anyone other than the patient, even someone undergoing treatment with informed consent. The huge costs of malpractice insurance reflect to some extent greed, the surplus of lawyers, and the sympathy of juries. But that sympathy in turn reflects unreasonable expectations that are not entirely the outcome of overselling the accomplishments of modern medicine and the magical powers of M.D.s. One result is the practice of defensive medicine: excessive testing and treatment to minimize the risks of malpractice suits and their success, incidentally increasing the incomes of M.D.s and hospitals.

On the whole, uncertainty aversion, whether by individuals, M.D.s, or firms, retards technological progress and is harmful to health from a social rather than individual point of view. Since technological progress is one cause of the great increase in health care costs, it could slow that increase. But the risk-prone attitude of the sick, eager to try anything new without considering the superiority of the new technology to existing alternatives, encourages technological change and raises costs. Much depends on the specific technology: Does it extend the scope of medical care? Does it keep sick people alive by receiving care continuously without cure, or does it eliminate the need for further medical care? Does the new technology reduce the costs of treatment, as did penicillin and smallpox vaccination, or does it increase them, as does cardiac surgery?

Attitudes toward risk and uncertainty are quite different when the patient is desperate, feeling that there is little to lose from experimental and danger-ous therapies. We see this in the FDA's bowing to pressure from the AIDS lobby to accelerate approval of drugs known to be dangerous, whose effec-tiveness is unproven, to accept "quarter-way" technologies. Experimental drugs have long been available for treating patients who otherwise would die, but only under carefully controlled conditions.

Risk aversion is at odds with the American character, which is still alive. I doubt that it is a major contributor to excessive demand. We cannot say that demand for medical services is greater here than in other advanced countries. Americans visit doctors less often, but lack of full coverage and shortage of general practitioners are factors. Americans take fewer pills than the Japanese or Germans, although again cost may be a factor. There are too many differences between systems to draw any assured conclusions.

In other areas, there is much evidence of a greater willingness to take risks. Americans are more willing to change jobs and careers, readier to move to other cities and regions. Their supply of entrepreneurs and venture capital cannot be matched.

Risk aversion that leads to excessive demand for medical services is also present in the field of public health: demands for environmental safety, which sometimes border on the absurd. Many years ago it was discovered that swordfish had a high concentration of mercury, and for a time no swordfish was eaten. Mercury in fish is probably true of nearly all large fish, certainly of tuna, which are long-lived and second only to man on the food chain. That is now forgotten. Then there is the fear of radon emission, which is found wherever granite is found, in stone foun-dations, in curbstones, in gravel used in roadbuilding, in Denver. The electromagnetic field (EMF) is back in fashion. Where shall we place all the high-voltage transmission lines? It is time for a return of concern about carcinogenic aflatoxin in peanuts, corn. The public can worry about only one or two threats at a time. There are many more. In some cases there may be real cause for concern and then it becomes part of the agenda of the FDA or the EPA or OSHA. Most of the time, the concerns are passing fads, which may do much damage to particular industries and generate lobbies and support industries of their own, adding to pub-lic health costs.

Risk aversion and excessive demand for environmental safety are ex-pressed more in "social" or political demand than in individual demand, as is the case with medical care. Such demand results in even more unbalanced results: spending millions to avert a single death here, hundreds to avert another death somewhere else. It is discussed briefly in Chapter 11.

The Rejection of Disability

The Middle Ages had its beggars, who performed the essential moral function of providing others with the opportunity for alms, thereby facilitating
their sojourn through Purgatory to the Pearly Gates. Our age must have its
disabled, its handicapped. In a meritocratic society, driven by the performance principle, compassion and guilt are targeted on those who do not
make the grade. Every handicap must be abolished. (But in a society where
the concept of performance and achievement is relative, there will always
be the handicapped.) Should the handicapped learn how to surmount or
circumvent their deficiencies, how to cope, they would relieve "society" of
its responsibility to succor them. We spend billions on saving "preemies"
doomed to a short and miserable life, on organ transplants requiring lifelong
medication to suppress the immune system and guarantee repeated infections, on reconstructive surgery for the malformed, on procedures to restore
hearing or sight or to correct mental defects. Since in fact many handicaps
are irremediable by medical means, at any cost, then we proceed to alter the
environment at any cost so that the condition will no longer constitute a
handicap (we also strive to eliminate the word "handicap" from the English
language; it is now "physically challenged"). Many billions have been spent
on ramps everywhere, on specially equipped buses, to provide mobility for
the lame, the paralyzed. It could have been accomplished more conveniently and at much lower cost by radio cabs on call were it not for the
attitude that disability is to be abolished, not to be assisted. By this approach we try to avoid discrediting people's ability to cope and affronting
their dignity and self-esteem. These are consequences of the medicalization
of life, the degradation of individual responsibility. I am not suggesting that
nothing should be done if there is no effective medical treatment, but sometimes we go too far.

The Denial of Death

Cultural views on death have changed radically. Until recently, death was
certain and arrived at a fixed time for everyone. Now, there is no natural
death. It is the task of the M.D. to prolong life, to frustrate death.[15] There
has been a great change in attitude toward death, an unwillngness to accept
its inevitability, a refusal to face it with grace.[16] This change was no doubt
influenced by the spectacular advances in medical technology since World
War II. I illustrate it in terms of our experience with war and its victims.
The Civil War resulted in more deaths than all subsequent wars combined,
from a much smaller population. There was no hiding the casualties or the

suffering. Yet the war went on to its military conclusion. Many men were gassed in World War I, but we carried on. World War II resulted in nearly seven times as many deaths as any war since, yet no one called for its premature cessation. The Vietnam war, in the eye of television, was carried on for years in the face of much public opposition. A few casualties in Somalia, and the world's greatest military power (?) tucks its tail between its legs and beats a frantic retreat. Now we are told that there will be no foreign intervention that places a single soldier's life at risk. (What are soldiers for? Let us hope our local police forces do not follow suit.) Consider the treatment of casualties: those wounded in World War II received treatment and service-connected disability compensation proportionate to their injuries. Vietnam victims of Agent Orange, a clearly pathogenic chemical, went through years of debate on its effects. But Persian Gulf War veterans, all volunteers (unlike most who served in Vietnam), complaining of a variety of ailments, real and imagined, slight and serious, none of which have been connected so far in any way to their experience there, have already been given free medical care and compensation based solely on the initial date of incidence of their complaint within one year, or perhaps two, of their service in the Gulf. Whoever heard of the missing-in-action (MIA) issue after World War II, or even after the Korean war, which had many more MIAs than Vietnam? Now the issue will not die, although any MIAs who are still living must be happy with their Vietnamese families and have no intention of returning, and though most MIAs will remain so forever. A pathological fear of death, an unwillingness to accept consequences. It is not just the availability of new technology that might stave off death, or prolong life, that results in demands for extraordinary measures at great cost. People do not love life more, or grieve more for the dead; there has been a sea change in attitudes toward death. The sense of immortality that is the province of the young has pervaded all age groups.

Debates about the quality of life, conflicts between the needs and demands of the very old and the young, must sharpen as the number and proportion of the very old increase. Already, one-third of all Medicare dollars are spent on patients in their last year of life. For the irreversible (to our present knowledge) and degenerative diseases of the old, all that medical progress can be expected to accomplish is to protract the process and raise the costs. But we cannot attribute the increased expenditures to the availability of new technologies alone; there must be motivation also, the observed obsession with health and life that leads people to allow, even induce, the health care industry to concentrate on the postponement of the inevitable rather than the quality of life. Is this obsession rational? Must we as citizens, taxpayers, and purchasers of health insurance tolerate our mutual obsession? Although this is discussed under excessive demand, it could also be discussed under oversupply, since both sides bear responsibility.

The Medicalization of Morality

Biological evolution has been described as a process of foetalization.[17] This process has now become social. The independent, self-sufficient individual of the nineteenth century has been transformed into a ward of "society," in turn a ward of the state. No one can be expected to cope with his or her own handicaps; no one is expected to cope with others'. Addiction and overindulgence are no longer crimes or sins but sickness. Much crime has been redefined as sickness; theft is kleptomania, if not justified redistribution; arson is pyromania. A search is on for drugs to reduce the craving for crack or cocaine, and some drugs are already available for alcoholics and other habit-ridden folks. Criminals of all sorts are not to be punished or stopped from further criminal behavior but are to be understood and treated.

The ills and sins of children are visited on their parents—the children were unloved or overdoted, given undue responsibility, neglected, toilet-trained too young, torn between indulgent and disciplinarian parents, or abused. We are all victims. The wonder of it is that we are not all criminals or mentally disturbed. Is *perestroika* the result of the discontinuance of swaddling in Russia? of central heating? Whether we blame parents (who must themselves be the victims of their early history) or that abstract collective noun "society," this attitude represents an abdication of responsibility by the individual (or of the child, in the case of parents prepared to assume all "blame") for one's own condition and for changing that condition, a dependence on outside agents, whether government intervention or medical treatment. The medicalization of society is but one aspect of the socialization of morality.

The evident unwillingness of millions to do what they obviously know ought to be done to preserve their health—stop smoking, change life habits of diet and exercise, avoid stress—has numerous explanations. But among them are the wide acceptance of conflicting ideologies:

1. We are all victims; our behavior is conditioned if not determined by childhood experiences; we are not responsible. This appears to be a major philosophy of psychotherapy and criminal justice.
2. Everything is in our genes, which leads to a blame-free "criminal" justice system and predisposes if not determines health outcomes, whether these result from ostensibly voluntary behavior (drug addiction, alcoholism) or from involuntary responses of the body to normal

environment (allergies, diabetes) or from internal breakdown of body functions (Alzheimer's).

3. Anyone can do anything, be anything—the prevailing educational philosophy. It also drives many health nuts, joggers, and presidential aspirants. It shares with traditional philosophy the belief that it is up to us, that outcomes are an individual responsibility.

I sense that the balance has shifted toward the default of individual responsibility. We, as citizens, taxpayers, and insurance premium payers, tolerate the consequences of such behavior, even encourage it by paying the bill.

Demographics and Social Structure

The need for, demand for, institutional treatment and care depends on social structure as well as medical indications. Many cases that could be treated at home, if there were other adult members of the family to provide care, require hospitalization in single-person or single-adult family units, or even in family units with more than one capable adult when all healthy adults are employed away from home. It is not just the prevalence of the nuclear family and now the single-parent family and increased female labor-force participation that have reduced capacity for home care and treatment, it is the separation of home and workplace associated with the decline of agriculture and the urbanization and metropolization of the nation. This process is now over. But changes in age of marriage, in living arrangements of unmarried adults, in metropolitan patterns of residence, in residential mobility, in local community organization in large cities—all can change needs for institutional care. The care of sick children when parents work outside the home (and the care of healthy children when the single parent is hospitalized) remains a problem without a solution in many communities. Much of the increased demand for medical services resulting from these demographic changes cannot be labeled excessive demand, although were it not for insurance coverage, there would be much less of it.

Rationing

With health care insurance, there will always be complaints of delays, denials. As long as health care is free, too much will be demanded; the supply of health care providers and facilities required to meet all demands will be excessive and far too costly. The public is becoming more knowledgeable, more critical, more demanding of quality health care. The prevalence of third-party payments reduces the role of quality rationing by price, so everyone wants the best.

Americans, many of them, believe that they are entitled to the best health care. But this is impossible; only a few can get the best. Suppose we all agree that the Smith-Jones Clinic is the best. Then ten times as many customers demand access as the clinic can handle. What to do? The clinic could raise its prices sky-high, eliminating most customers. This is rationing by price, which we reject. Or it could pick those it thinks have most to benefit (perhaps excluding anyone over age sixty-five) or pick blindly by lottery. It is still rationing, but not by price. Or it could expand its capacity tenfold. Then its quality would have to fall, it would no longer be considered the best, and other clinics would be faced with the problem of rationing excessive demand. Not everyone can get above-average anything.

Why do beneficaries always want more than any viable system can deliver? First, of course, they are unaware of their costs, or if aware, the cost to them of additional services may approach zero. Second, there are exaggerated expectations of what medical care can deliver, largely induced by the medical care establishment. Third, there is the change in what many people consider acceptable states of health and well-being; ours has become a hypochondriac society, in part because of the enhanced ability to deliver effective services and propaganda to that effect, in part because of rising incomes and an increased ability to pay for health care. Fourth, we have experienced a correlated shift in self-concepts from the Calvinistic, tough image of the past to a self-indulgent, tender image of the present, and a related change from a concept of health and sickness as natural outcomes of personal behavior, mental attitude, and uncontrollable events to one of medical interventionism, victimology, and extroversion of responsibility. Related to this change toward a narcissistic self-image is an increase in risk aversion and a demand for a fail-safe, risk-free life and an extreme reluctance to accept death as inevitable, a pathological fear of death. The demand for fail-safe cures is part of the explanation not only for the large increase in malpractice suits but for the preposterous awards recommended by juries.

Notes

1. David Reisman, *Market and Health* (New York: St. Martin's Press, 1993), 25.

2. Don Kenkel, "Consumer Health Information and Demand for Medical Care," *Review of Economics and Statistics* 72 (November 1990): 587–95.

3. Milford Rouse, Inaugural Address as President of the AMA, *Journal of the American Medical Association* 258 (July 17, 1967): 87–89.

4. A.J. Culyer and Adam Wagstaff, "Equity and Equality in Health and Health Care," *Journal of Health Economics* 12 (1993): 431–57.

5. Cited in Daniel Callahan, *What Kind of Life: The Limits of Medical Progress* (New York: Simon and Schuster, 1990), 84.

6. Edmund Pellegrino, "The Sociocultural Impact of Twentieth Century Therapeutics," in *The Therapeutic Revolution: Essays in the Social History of American Medicine,* ed. Morris Vogel and Charles Rosenberg, 245–66, esp. 262 (Philadelphia: University of Pennsylvania Press, 1979).

7. Daniel Callahan, "Health and Society: Some Ethical Imperatives," in *Doing Better and Feeling Worse: Health in the United States,* ed. John H. Knowles, 22–33, esp. 28 (New York: Norton, 1977).

8. Lewis Thomas, "On the Science and Technology of Medicine," in *Doing Better and Feeling Worse: Health in the United States,* ed. John Knowles, 35–46 (New York: Norton, 1977).

9. Stanley Wohl, *The Medical Industrial Complex* (New York: Harmony Books, 1984), 61.

10. Victor Fuchs, *Who Shall Live?* (New York: Basic Books, 1974), 27.

11. Rene Fox, "The Medicalization and Demedicalization of American Society," in *Doing Better and Feeling Worse: Health in the United States,* ed. John Knowles, 9–22 (New York: Norton, 1977).

12. Ivan Illich, *Medical Nemesis: The Expropriation of Health* (New York: Bantam Books, 1976), 112.

13. U.S. Department of Health and Human Services, *Health United States* (Washington, D.C.: Government Printing Office, 1993), 153; see also earlier editions.

14. Victor Fuchs, *The Health Economy* (Cambridge, Mass.: Harvard University Press, 1986), 43–44, 239–40.

15. Rick J. Carlson, *The End of Medicine* (New York: Wiley, 1975), 177.

16. Yair Aharoni, *The No-Risk Society* (Chatham, N.J.: Chatham House, 1981), 60.

17. George Annas, "Informed Consent, Cancer and Truth in Prognosis," *New England Journal of Medicine* 330 (January 20, 1994): 223–25.

18. Loren Eiseley, *The Immense Journey* (New York: Vintage Books, 1957), 130.

9

Research and Technology

Changing Concepts of Disease

Modern health care could be said to date from the development of a small-pox vaccine by Edward Jenner in 1796, although vaccines did not become an important part of public health until the twentieth century. The scientific base for the "germ theory of disease," which has been a central part of medical thinking and practice, was laid by Louis Pasteur and Robert Koch in the nineteenth century with the discovery of bacteria. The same discovery gave an added impetus to public health measures improving the quality of water supplies and providing for waste disposal, although these practices had been known to reduce illness for a very long time. Although the first antibiotic was discovered in the nineteenth century, and penicillin in 1929, the antibiotic revolution that provided the therapeutic as distinguished from the preventive implementation of Pasteur's findings did not really start until around 1940. Since then, it has largely run its course, as microorganisms have developed resistance to most antibiotics. Staphylococcus, pneumococcus, and tuberculin bacilli have become resistant to almost all antibiotics. Although new vaccines against malaria, hepatitis B, and venereal diseases perhaps remain to be developed, and drugs effective against viruses are in their infancy, the simple germ model of disease has nearly exhausted its potential. Its very success has pushed cancer and cardiovascular diseases to the top of the medical agenda. Newer, more complex models are evolving.

The simple causal germ model, focusing on an external prime and proximate cause, is not adequate even where the germ theory has been established as sufficient and necessary cause. It is not a question of replacing a bad model with a better one, but of supplementing, modifying a model that has proven very useful and will so remain, to improve our understanding where the germ theory is inadequate, in particular where it appears to be irrelevant. We have no reason to believe that all forms of diabetes or astigmatism are caused by microorganisms or by any external agency.

Two new models, neither entirely new nor separable, are the genetic model and the immunological model. A fourth is the environmental or behavioral model. The role of inheritance in predisposing to illness, and the role of resistance, inherited or acquired, to particular ailments has long been recognized. Hemophilia has played a prominent role in the descent of kings. Kings and other prominent persons have long been provided resistance to arsenic and various poisons by taking small gradually increasing doses. But until recently, neither the scientific understanding of processes of genetic and immunological vulnerabilities and resistances nor the techniques required to find out were in existence.

There are some diseases that people are born with or, because of their DNA, will develop (e.g., Down's syndrome and Parkinson's disease). In other diseases, we are born with a predisposition to them by our genetic inheritance (many cancers, some mental illnesses). Disease states may be triggered by environmental or behavioral conditions such as diet, stress. We are born with a wide variety of somatic and psychosomatic responses and a wide range of abilities to cope with disease. As we continue to decipher the genetic code, we may pinpoint the role of heredity and learn how to forestall its consequences.

The immunological model of disease may well have a mainly genetic underlying basis. There is evidence of psychological influence on the immune system as well.[1] To what extent does the body muster adequate defenses against external assault? How does it learn to distinguish between its own and foreign matter, how does it remember previous invasions through the process of immunization, how can it be taught to forget, when the foreign invader is an organ transplant or an antibiotic? How can learning disabilities be prevented or corrected when the body becomes vulnerable to internal attack because it mistakenly identifies its own cells as foreign or cannot distinguish between its own and foreign (cancer, bacteria) cells? How can the body's defense department and its FBI be strengthened and kept on target?

We have learned of the contribution of fluoride to reducing dental caries, of calcium in preventing osteoporosis, and the role of many other chemicals in diet and environment to disease and its prevention. On the other hand, some cancers have increased, and some environmental carcinogens have been identified and a search goes on for others—pesticides, industrial chemicals. Some diseases perhaps cannot be understood except through all four models and must be dealt with in this quadripartite fashion. There is certainly a genetic component in the incidence of most kinds of cancer. There is viral involvement in some. There are environmental factors. And there are immunological factors as well. Prevention or treatment may proceed through the development of vaccines *and* modifying the immune system *and* genetic research and counseling—and, in the future, therapy *and* environmental controls. These diverse perspectives on health and illness should determine the direction of research.

Medicine is an art, not a science, not because of a lack of scientific knowledge or content but because of the idiosyncratic character of the patient. The M.D. is concerned with identifying and coping with the unique characteristics of each patient, whereas the medical scientist-researcher is concerned with the common elements in the development, behavior, and responses of many individuals. One focuses on the differences, the other on the commonalities, even though both deal with the same range of phenomena. Research and treatment are separate undertakings. An exchange of information between them is necessary and works well enough from research to the practice of medicine. But the observations of the healers are not systematically collected for the benefit of the researchers.

How Much Research?

Much biomedical research is financed, and some of it is conducted, by the federal government. This is the research that private for-profit firms do not conduct and yet should be conducted. Much of government-financed research is basic research—the foundation for much of the applied research conducted by firms, of great potential social benefit. Since the results of basic research may not be patentable or marketable, for they still require applied research to produce marketable products, private firms have not conducted it. The situation is changing, as the distinction between basic and applied research becomes fuzzy, as the time lag shortens, as firms in some areas must conduct some of the basic research in order to perfect marketable products. Until the early 1980s, the federal government financed more than half of all biomedical research, twice as much as industry. The situation has changed dramatically, as industry now spends more than the federal government (Table 9.1).

A second type of research not performed by private firms without public incentives is research whose economic returns are too small to cover the cost of research and development (R&D) and production. This may be the case because there are few beneficiaries (so-called orphan drugs, defined as having fewer than 200,000 potential users); because the beneficiaries have a limited ability to pay (river blindness in Africa, Chagas disease in Brazil); or because much of the benefit accrues not to the individuals treated but to others, even society at large (preventive technologies).

Table 9.1

Trends in Health Research
(in millions of dollars)

	Total	Federal	Industry	State/Local	Nonprofits
1960	$ 886	$ 448	$ 253	$ 46	$ 139
1970	2,847	1,667	795	170	215
1980	7,899	4,725	2,459	480	313
1992	28,717	11,727	13,870	1,900	1,221

Source: U.S. Department of Health and Human Services, *Health United States* (Washington, D.C.: Government Printing Office, 1993), table 141.

The share of medical costs allocated to research and development is less than 4 percent. These numbers per se mean nothing because research is not conducted, or its products used, in a one-to-one relationship, as is true of medical diagnosis and treatment. Research, unlike treatment, does not increase in total costs as the population increases or ages. The cost of developing a new drug is the same whatever the size of the market. The incentive to develop it, however, depends on prospective market size, perhaps one reason why the United States does more than its share of medical R&D and has contributed about half of all new drugs in the past half century.

How much should be spent depends on the research agenda and its requirements, nothing else. Changing directions of research imply changing manpower requirements. As we learned during the 1960s space race, spending more money means nothing without the highly talented and trained manpower to go with it, and it takes eight to ten years to expand the supply of such manpower. The proportion of M.D.s employed as researchers has declined, but they are on the whole not as well trained for this purpose as Ph.D.s in relevant fields. The large and widening gap in earnings between Ph.D.s and practicing M.D.s guarantees a declining supply of M.D.s for research and helps keep down the cost of research. Fortunately, we can draw on rare talent from many other countries. Look at the list of authors in almost any technical journal in this country; a high proportion are foreign visitors and immigrants in our leading research centers.

If there is any reason to worry that research spending has not kept up with research opportunities, it is that the costs of developing new products, drugs in particular, have risen much more than the costs of medical care, and hence the output of new products has declined; meanwhile, the scope of what is considered illness requiring health care has greatly widened.

Much concern is expressed that technological advance will be slowed by efforts to contain the costs of health care. Since R&D accounts for less than 4 percent of health care costs, it is hardly a priority area for cost cutting, apart from the fact that industry alone contributes half the total. It is the direction of research, not its total cost, that needs to change.

Many tests and procedures are overused, and reducing their frequency would reduce demand for the appropriate tools and supplies. The research area that has the most to fear from an effective containment of medical costs is that of very expensive equipment, such as MRIs, each of which must be used by many people if they are to cover their cost. There are far too many such instruments to provide for legitimate needs—over 2,900 of them. A reduction in their number, or a drastic decline in new demand for such instruments, could reduce their profitability sufficiently to discourage some research into their improvement, replacement, or research into other similarly expensive instruments. Some drugs also are greatly overused, and should there be substantial reduction in their prescription and sale, the prospective market for improvements and replacements would also be reduced.

The application and the extensive use (some would say, overuse or premature use) of the results of research are another matter. The prospect that new drugs and procedures will not be used as soon or as often as in the past, that FDA approval may be more difficult to obtain, that public subsidies for their use will be reduced, that insurance coverage will be delayed or denied, may indeed give pharmaceutical and medical equipment firms some thought. The prospect that public funds for R&D will be better allocated in terms of prospective payoff, cutting off some medical schools and universities and foundations, may worry producers and grant recipients.

Everything human beings can discover will be discovered; everything we can invent will be invented. The question is, when, at what cost? As to research, no one can say in advance what is enough, what is too much. The output is unknown and the probability of a successful output is unknown; the cost and time required for success are unknown. That is one reason why spending on research is so vulnerable to political pressures, to interest-group influence.

Such pressures lead to premature efforts at applied research when basic research needs to be done first; at trying to develop a cure before we understand the disease. The war on cancer of the 1960s was a political initiative, an example of premature and largely wasted effort. The current war on AIDS, going on for ten years with minimal progress in treatment or medical prevention, bears all the earmarks of another failed political crusade. Both diverted a significant share of government spending and highly qualified personnel from research in other, perhaps more promising, areas.

But to repeat, one only knows the value of research ex post facto. How much research depends on scientific opportunities for technological breakthroughs of value to human life and health. But such opportunities are created, not given; hence, how much research has been done helps determine how much should be done, and what kinds.

The case is not for less R&D or for more R&D. Partly it is for a redirection of R&D toward areas of great potential payoff. But mainly it is a case for avoiding the premature introduction of new products and processes into the marketplace, where they are inevitably overused, even misused. "Premature" means before it is clearly established that the products confer significant net benefits not previously available or are a significant improvement over existing products or procedures. And there's the rub. How does one determine this without trying it out on adequate (often large) numbers of patients over a long time period? Probably one cannot; but one can keep it experimental, not let it seep into the commercial market until significant net gains are verified. This restraint runs counter to the interests of researchers, of manufacturers, of M.D.s driven by the technological imperative, of patients desperate for a technological fix. How does one distinguish between a "halfway" technology, which makes a little, or perhaps not even a little, difference, at great cost, siphoning resources away from more beneficial uses, and a "breakthrough" technology? The FDA deemed that of the 348 drugs introduced by the twenty-five largest manufacturers between 1981 and 1988 only 12 were important therapeutic advances; 44 had modest potential for gains.[2] Perhaps most of the other 292 should not have been introduced at all.

Not all halfway technologies, which neither prevent nor cure, are a waste of research and medical resources. Insulin for diabetes is a case in point; it can save some lives, improve the quality of many more, while research goes on. Kidney dialysis can be justified if it keeps a patient alive while waiting for a kidney transplant; otherwise, it is questionable. The suicide rate of those undergoing dialysis is reported to be 100 times the average. New drugs for mental illness make patients manageable and improve the quality of life of many more. On the other hand, medication to lower serum cholesterol in the expectation that it will lower the probability of a heart attack does not even treat a symptom but a characteristic somehow weakly correlated with incidence of heart attacks, whose reduction involves billions of dollars per year with risks of serious side effects and little benefit.

Why should the United States do the bulk of the basic and much of the applied R&D and then sell pharmaceuticals and other products to other countries that did not pay for their development at lower, often much lower, prices than charged at home? The American customer pays for most of the basic research via taxation and tax subsidies, ends up paying for the applied R&D via high prices, and contributes the bulk of the profits to pharmaceutical firms that for many years were at or near the top profit makers in American industry. The rest of the world gets a free ride. They get access to new drugs, often before they are available for sale in the United States, and get them at lower, often much lower, prices. If other countries did a larger share of the R&D, we too would benefit from the availability of the resulting research products, even though we would not pay a lower but surely a higher price than the customers in the country of origin.

Research is a large part of the problem of excessive and escalating health care costs; it is also a large part of the solution. It can concentrate on cures that cut costs of illness and ways of preventing illness in the first place, or it can pour forth halfway technologies that neither prevent nor cure at great cost. Much depends on the FDA. It has concentrated unduly on safety, which can be determined conclusively only through prolonged use by humans, not enough on assuring that new products it approves are not only effective but are significantly more effective than products already available or significantly less dangerous. Procedures are not subject to FDA approval; they can be introduced and widely used without the equivalent assurance that they are significantly better or safer than existing alternatives. Then research becomes part of the problem, not of the solution.

It makes more sense to arrive at a research budget from the bottom up rather than the top down: what are the promising and urgent research projects, and how much in human and financial resources is required to conduct them? Ordering projects by priority, one arrives at a total not given in advance. Of course, some limit must be imposed, whether set by a firm's financial capability or by whatever budget is approved by Congress and the president. The criteria for choosing projects and setting limits differ: the firm considers the prospect of marketable products and the income derived from them, whereas the government's research agenda and budget are set to a considerable extent by political pressures, to some extent by scientific interest and prospects.

What Kind of Research?

Research resources must be allocated in complex ways. What illness should be stressed? Research personnel is limited, even if financial resources were not. How shall a selected disease be addressed? Improved ability to diagnose? Improved treatment? Ability to prevent?[3] The reader is likely to think, prevention of course! How we wish that were possible in every case. It may be a very long time, possibly never, before we learn how to prevent most cancers, never mind the common cold. Thus a judgment of technical feasibility is involved in allocating research resources. But for those who think that the impossible just takes a little longer, another consideration is the time frame: how much longer? Are we prepared to put off final success for decades, generations, rather than focus on some palliative in the near future? Is the search for a preventive, or a cure, premature? Does the current state of knowledge justify elaborate tests of thousands of substances, or should we first gain a better understanding of what is going on in the afflicted body?

The current system of compensation through third-party reimbursement has biased research and development in the direction of product-adding rather than cost-reducing innovation, a direction that tends to inflate medical costs by expanding the scope of treatment and by substituting high-cost procedures and drugs for marginally less effective but cheaper alternatives. This bias needs to be countered, in part by reducing the acceptance of "halfway" technologies. Perhaps it is not possible or advisable to withdraw FDA approval already granted, but future approval could be contingent on significant improvement over existing alternatives. As a second line of defense, it is certainly possible for third-party payers to deny reimbursement. HMOs are in the best position to limit the use of costly new drugs of questionable superiority. Medicare compensation based on diagnosis-related groups (DRGs) is a blunter instrument toward cost reduction. Truly new products could be cost cutting, whereas me-too products are usually more expensive and hardly more effective than their competitors.

Applied research may yield a preventive or a treatment for a particular ailment. Basic research may shed light on many ailments. Efforts to come up with drugs to cure AIDS, or vaccines to prevent it, have failed so far. But the basic research on viruses that the disease and the failure to come up with an immediate cure or preventive have stimulated may shed light on other viruses, may eventually lead to better vaccines and drugs for many of them. Basic research has spillover benefits normally lacking in applied research. But it takes patience; the payoff is indirect, and takes much time. One problem is that private firms, whose interest is in salable products, now account for half of all biomedical research. Another is that political pressures are biasing the federal government's contribution to research toward quick fixes, applied research, depriving basic research not only of funds but of rare talent.

The bias toward new drugs and procedures by both suppliers and consumers, supported by third-party payments, means increased use of drugs and procedures early in the learning curve. Premature adoption means higher costs, greater risks, and less benefit than would a slower, less rash adoption.

Taking a long view, the great breakthroughs early in this century—vaccination, public health measures, antibiotics—led to much of the more recent large increases in medical costs. They largely eliminated diseases that were self-limiting if not promptly fatal, which afflicted primarily the young, leading to large increases in life expectancy. The three main causes of death in the early and middle adult years are now accidents, homicide, and AIDS. The first two are not part of the medical agenda at all (although emergency medicine saves more of the lives formerly lost as a result), but public health concerns. AIDS, because of the behavioral nature of its acquisition and spread, is also a public health concern, since there are no medical means of preventing or curing it today, nor are there likely to be for a long time; nevertheless, it incurs large and increasing medical costs. Research on behavioral illness and accidents is always relatively neglected because it produces intangible knowledge, not marketable products.

Third-party payments and changing age distribution have reallocated R&D activities toward the conditions afflicting the elderly, illnesses that are not self-limiting, that may be fatal, but often only after years of suffering and treatment; for example, cancer, heart and vascular problems, Alzheimer's, osteoporosis, arthritis. Even successful treatment confers smaller benefits to the elderly and to their dependents because of the shorter remaining lifetime. It is estimated that the total elimination of cancer, for instance, would raise life expectancy less than two years. Research is properly concentrated on these not new but newly dominant health problems. But Philip Abelson is concerned that "research and care [are] focused too strongly on cardiovascular diseases and cancer and on using medicine and technology to prolong burdensome and meaningless existence."[4] Should we learn to prevent some of these diseases, or cure them, there would be large gains in quality of life, modest gains in life expectancy, perhaps substantial savings in health care costs, since even though our ability to treat them is limited, much money is spent on them. What happens after, no one knows; what will be the dominant ailments, or causes of death, should we ever be able to prevent cancer and cardiovascular disease?

One might favor research benefiting the young and those of working age, with a long potential life expectancy, who may have dependents, and whose work in itself may generate externalities, rather than research primarily of benefit to the retired. But that is a question of values.

If the human life span is limited, as we have every reason to believe, new research breakthroughs in the diseases primarily affecting the elderly must lead to rapidly diminishing returns. If the gains in life expectancy between 1900 and 1950, from 47.3 to 68.2, were to be repeated, the average life expectancy would rise to 89.1 in the year 2000. We might reach 78 years.

Countries such as Japan may be approaching the feasible limit to average life expectancy.[5] Until science finds some way of extending the normal life span, research on the ailments of the old must come at increasing costs and diminishing returns. It is time to think less about saving lives or postponing death—there is less and less to gain in that direction—and more about improving the quality of life. The area of mental health is underfunded, perhaps because so much of the expected outcome is knowledge, not products, perhaps because mental illness is poorly covered by insurance, limiting the market for new products. But these concerns should not apply to federal funding. In 1986, although schizophrenics occupied 40 percent of all long-term hospital beds, and direct care costs were $36 billion, federal research spending per patient was $14 for schizophrenia, $10 for depression, but $130 for heart problems and $10,000 for muscular dystrophy.[6]

One may question whether R&D should be devoted to orphan drugs (defined in the United States as drugs for diseases afflicting fewer than 200,000 people) instead of to treatments for diseases with many sufferers; whether funds should be allocated to beneficiary groups that cannot pay, even though benefits are large, if it means diversion of resources from developing treatments for beneficiaries who can pay. A market of 200,000 does not seem that small; it is the exorbitant cost of developing new drugs that make it an "orphan"; more effort should be directed toward revising regulations in order to reduce that cost. On the one hand, we make the development of these drugs uneconomic; on the other, we pay taxes to provide subsidies for their development. Where to cut off depends on total public resources made available for research.

Research Needs and Opportunities

One may distinguish between research needs and research opportunities. Needs are current, often pressing. Opportunities can wait, if necessary, with little harm done. Some research is necessary not to advance our ability to improve health and save lives but merely to stand still. Progress is proving temporary in some cases, as antibiotics lose their effectiveness. Bacteria acquire resistance. Vaccines lose their effectiveness. So not conducting research is not an option. Trying to predict research breakthroughs and their impact on quality of life, life expectancy, and costs of medical care is a foolhardy undertaking. I do any attempt any "gee whiz" crystal balling, only a brief listing of important research efforts under way.

The first priority is to overcome the technological obsolescence of existing treatments. Many microorganisms have demonstrated an uncanny ability to evolve resistance to existing antibiotics and other drugs and to the immunities generated by existing vaccines. The great antibiotic revolution of midcentury was only a temporary victory. Research must continue. There is no truce in the war against microorganisms.

Pneumonia, once known as the "old man's friend," a quick death rather than prolonged suffering, is back; so is tuberculosis, which in some cases has developed resistance to all available drugs. Some strains of golden staph resist most known antibiotics; only vancomycin is fully effective, and for how long we do not know. Salmonella and gonorrhea are resistant to penicillin. This problem, strains of microbes that through Darwinian natural selection resist antibiotics, is very worrisome. Perhaps it would have been slowed by the more judicious use of antibiotics, but it would have arisen in any case. Research does not appear to be staying ahead by developing new antibacterial agents. Development of new drugs to replace them is a high priority.[7]

The same problem of technological obsolescence found in antibiotics and other medicines has arisen in preventive treatment. Old vaccines are becoming less and less effective as new strains of microorganisms evolve and multiply. Even new vaccines may offer only partial protection for bacteria and viruses that come in many strains. For pneumonia, new vaccines protect against as many as twenty-three strains; they are only about 75 percent effective for adults, for there are over eighty strains, and new ones yet to develop or be discovered.[8] The annual flu vaccine protects against two or three of the most likely and/or most dangerous varieties, but there are others against which it offers no protection. Multiple strains, and the ability to develop new ones rapidly, is an unsurmounted problem in trying to develop a preventive vaccine against AIDS, which is more variable than influenza. Worldwide, malaria is the greatest killer disease; the plasmodium has in many cases developed resistance to most medications, and the mosquito vector in turn has developed resistance to insecticides. In advanced countries, an AIDS vaccine has higher priority, but whether at this time research should stress its development, before learning more about how to cope with viruses, is debatable. The most urgently needed vaccines in the developed world are for HIV, respiratory syncytial virus, and pneumococcus; whereas in the developing world, they are for malaria, tuberculosis, and again HIV.[9] Improved vaccines are needed also for measles and chicken pox. Work is in progress on improved cholera vaccines, on new vaccines for respiratory viruses, rotavirus (the cause of often fatal diarrhea in children in developing nations), and other viruses and bacteria.

The antibiotic revolution devastated bacteria but left viruses almost unscathed. For protection against some viruses, we have depended exclusively on vaccines. It is no longer true that there are no treatments for viruses. Compounds offer partial protection against influenza and other respiratory diseases, as well as herpes.[10] But we still lack means of treating most viral infections. Absent immunization, the search must continue for substances that can cure viral infections. A new approach toward fighting disease is the development of vaccines as means of stimulating the immune system after infection. It is being tried for leprosy, herpes, tuberculosis, hepatitis, and AIDS and may offer promise for other infections.[11] New viruses, or newly virulent viruses, keep cropping up from time to time to which research must be devoted.[12]

The problem of protection is not just a technical-scientific one. The number of preschool children without protection has been soaring. Measles epidemics have reappeared. One problem is that of letting down one's guard, thinking that the risk has been eliminated. But another is the cost: a full series of childhood vaccines has increased from $23 to $244 over the past decade.[13]

Drugs are poisons. All of them generate unwelcome side effects among some of their users; some of these can be dangerous, even fatal. A major reason is that the doses we take are far too large. We want the drug to influence the heart, or a swollen and painful joint, or the lungs. But we cannot place the drug just where we want it to go. We take too much of it because perhaps only a small proportion of the drug goes where it belongs, the rest spreads throughout the body and generates unwanted and unwelcome symptoms. Special delivery systems for drugs are on the way. The immune system is capable of producing an enormous number of different monoclonal antibodies, cells that can seek out and stick to a specific alien molecule. If combined with toxins, they destroy that specific molecule; if combined with some prophylactic drug or chemical missing in the body, they can deliver it where needed to cure or correct. Recombinant DNA techniques (recently developed ability to identify and slice off desired sections from strands of DNA) for reproducing cell proteins will permit us to attach a drug to an appropriate monoclonal antibody, resulting in more effective treatment with smaller doses and fewer adverse effects.

That is the theory, but there are problems: the human monoclonal antibodies that target only a specific type of cell cannot be reproduced in large quantity, and they are short-lived outside the body. The methods of production involve immortalization of antibody-producing cells by splicing them with a cancerlike cell from mice, producing hybridoma cells that can be cloned to produce large quantities. But the human immune system recognizes them as alien and rejects them. The alien component is being minimized to avoid rejection while still retaining long life, thus permitting massive supplementation of the body's own supply of appropriate antibodies. There is also a problem of reduced effectiveness as compared to the natural human cells.

There is much promise and need for research on malfunctioning immune systems. For individuals undergoing organ or tissue transplants, or bone-marrow transplants, it is necessary to suppress the immune system, which is currently done with drugs, especially cyclosporin. This ability to suppress has a dangerous by-product, susceptibility to infection. Monoclonal antibodies specific for a particular microorganism need to be injected to counter the effect of immune suppression in case of infection.[14] Another objective is to stimulate the normal immune system to improve its performance in fighting infection. But the most important objective of research on the immune system is a cure for autoimmune diseases; the immune system of some individuals regards some of its own cells as alien, and sets out to destroy them. Autoimmune diseases include muscular dystrophy, myasthenia gravis, arthritis, and some forms of diabetes. This involves genetic therapy, the insertion of a noninfective virus carrying particular genes in the hope of eventually replacing the defective genes that bring about the autoimmune reaction.[15]

New vaccines and drugs, improved delivery systems, therapy for the immune system, all employ what is commonly called biotechnology, which involves manipulation of genetic materials. Molecular biologists have taken over much of the research-oriented pharmaceutical industry from traditional chemists. The most important application, however, in terms of both costs and consequences, is testing for and prevention of genetic determination of predisposition toward disease.

The germ model of disease is of declining importance in this country. In the longer run research resources should shift toward genetics, which offers prospects for both prevention and treatment of conditions not caused by microorganisms, as well as the prospect of coping with vulnerability to those that are. There is little question that the next revolution in medicine, already under way, is genetic medicine. Eventually, during the next century, it may prove more important, and more permanent, than the antibiotic revolution of this century. Genetic influence is ubiquitous.

The first step is to identify the diseases that have a major genetic basis. This is relatively easy for the few that are determined by a single gene, such as cystic fibrosis or Parkinson's disease. It is more difficult when the genetic influence amounts to a predisposition, not determination, or when the genetic influence is exerted by several and possibly even many genes. Yet much has already been learned. Genetic influence is important for autism, schizophrenia, Alzheimer's, major affective disorder (manic depression), idiopathic epilepsy, rheumatoid arthritis, and peptic ulcers but is modest for hypertension, ischemic heart disease, male alcoholism.[16] Some of this was suspected from studies of family histories and of identical twins long before techniques were available to confirm and quantify the influence.

The second step is to identify the genes conducive to a particular illness. This did not become possible until the 1980s. It was relatively simple to do when a single gene was involved and its influence was large. The earliest diseases traced to their genetic determinants were indeed those resulting from a single mutation. Now scientists are preoccupied with identifying multiple genetic mutations associated with particular diseases. It will be a long time and will take great effort to puzzle out the contribution of different genes and combinations of genes to vulnerability to particular diseases. More than 600 genes associated with disease have already been identified, more than 100 associated with cancers, and thousands of diseases with some genetic component.[17] The two leading killers, cancer and heart disease, involve a large number of genes. In a few cases—cancer of the breast, ovarian cancer, prostate cancer, and colon cancer—specific genetic defects have been identified that greatly increase the probability of their occurrence.

Alzheimer's disease and osteoporosis, each afflicting many of the elderly, may be easier. Genes have been identified predisposing for Alzheimer's, and for bone mass, itself related to osteoporosis.[18] But most successes so far refer to rare diseases caused by a single gene.

Locating chromosomes and genes is only part of the problem. Then the mutation within the gene responsible for predisposition must be identified. Once this is done, decisions have to be made about genetic screening: who gets screened, and for what? Already newborns are screened for relatively rare but extremely serious genetic defects: Down's syndrome, Tay-Sachs disease, Parkinson's disease, phenylketonuria, hypothyroidism (which can be easily identified), and the individual bearing the defective gene is almost certain to develop the disease, although in the last two cases it can be prevented through treatment if caught early. But in time we will be able to identify hundreds of genetic defects, most of them much more difficult to locate than the single-gene diseases for which we already test. And in most cases the possession of a particular defect in a gene only increases the probability of an illness, sometimes by not very much, and the illness may not be very severe and may perhaps be treatable. There are ethical issues; who should be tested, who should be told.[19] There are enormous economic issues—costs could rise into the hundreds of billions. Genetic preventive therapy—treatment to correct a single gene—is in the experimental stage.[20] The prospect of effective genetic therapy for diseases involving several or many genes lies in the remote future.[21]

The first therapeutic test was in 1990. NIH's Recombinant DNA Advisory Committee has approved sixty-five gene therapy experiments. Such therapy will greatly broaden the scope of medical care; many untreatable conditions will become preventable. Others that are treatable will become preventable. Economic and ethical issues are very important. Who should be treated, for what? A large percentage of the American people support treatment for genetic "defects," including 43 percent in a 1992 poll favoring gene therapy to improve heritable physical characteristics, 42 percent for improving intelligence; other traits mentioned most often were height and baldness.[22]

Finally, far in the future, is the prospect of modifying germ cells themselves so that a defect is eradicated not just from a single individual but from any progeny conceived thereafter. This is what many respondents in the poll mentioned earlier had in mind. We need not be concerned yet about who should get what germ cell therapy for what purposes, nor about the cost. Many have been thinking about the dominant ethical implications, and hoping that the day will never come when it becomes possible.[23] For whatever can be done is almost certain to be done.

There is much progress in diagnostic ability, in particular in noninvasive ability. Computerized tomography (CT) scanners and magnetic resonance imagers (MRIs) are prime examples of improvement in diagnostic ability. Other imagers (positron tomography and nuclear magnetic resonance imagers) permit the observation of processes rather than just structure, a movie so to speak. This type of instrument is constantly being improved. CT scanners can be a substitute for visual inspection of colons and bronchial tubes. These instruments are more than diagnostic tools; they can add to our knowledge of the working of the body and especially the brain, and the physiological aspects of mental illness. Work is in progress toward a noninvasive test for Alzheimer's.[24] Another significant diagnostic development is the use of monoclonal antibodies (MABs) to diagnose infections. Since each infective agent brings about a great increase in the MAB specific to it, and we can identify the MAB, we can pinpoint the cause of infection and determine the best course of treatment. In time we will be able to identify quickly any infectious microorganism.[25]

Materials research seeks to produce better materials to replace organic substances temporarily or permanently: skin substitutes, bone substitutes, blood cell and plasma substitutes, dental replacement materials, improved orthopedic and prosthetic materials and devices, vascular replacements, cardiovascular materials.[26] Work continues on artificial organs or partial replacements and devices assisting the operation of organs: hearts, livers, lungs.[27] A new area of research made possible by advances in microelectronics includes neural prostheses and devices, implantable electrodes, which may in time help restore sight and hearing and restore some motor control of paralyzed body parts.[28]

Why is research concentrated on illness and its cure, why so little on prevention, vaccines excepted? Particular illnesses can focus the minds of the public, whereas the search for environmental health hazards cannot. Illness and its treatment and cure are often concentrated in time, and in particular individuals, whereas environmental hazards and their prevention, and health-contributing individual behavior, are very long-term activities and make a statistical rather than a personal difference. But the main problem with research on the relationship between behavior and health is that the end product is a "public good" available to all without cost. That is why it must be financed by governments and nonprofits. As to research on the relationship between environment and health, again in most cases there is no end product that can be sold to individuals or to governments or business firms. Sulfur dioxide turns out to be unhealthy, so the EPA requires power plants to reduce their sulfur emissions. If they do this by using more expensive low-sulfur coal, the only firms to profit are low-sulfur coal mines. If they do it by installing stack scrubbers, firms that develop and manufacture stack scrubbers gain, but they are not the firms that do the research and demonstrate the harmful effects of sulfur emissions. Much search has been conducted for carcinogens in the environment; most changes in tumor cells are believed to arise after birth, the result of environmental factors.[29] But the search for neurotoxins has hardly begun.

Regulation and Pharmaceutical Research

Pharmaceuticals are one area in which the productivity of medical care has been rising, and often rapidly. New drugs are often more effective and/or have fewer side effects than the drugs they displace; some new drugs help treat conditions formerly untreatable. Prescription drugs are a small share of medical expenditures and their prices have declined relative to health costs over the long run (although since 1985 this trend may have been reversed). But prescription drugs are poorly covered by insurance, and costly ones are disproportionately consumed by the elderly, hence the concern. Better insurance coverage would increase the demand for them. There is also concern that pressures to reduce the price of drugs will have an adverse effect on R&D and the rate of progress in this area.

Regulation has played a major role in the supply and cost of drugs. The reaction to the thalidomide tragedy of 1961 was more traumatic in America than in Germany, where the drug was developed and most of the deformed babies were born, even though the drug was never introduced legally in this country. Requirements for effectiveness were first imposed in 1962 and those for safety tightened, greatly increasing the time and cost for FDA approval, cutting the rate of new drugs approved by around half and leading to increasing concentration in large multinational corporations.[30] Whereas 564 new drugs were approved in the decade before the 1962 regulations, only 166 were approved in the subsequent decade.[31] The tightened regulations also led to some shift of manufacture abroad, since exports required prior approval by the FDA.[32] Although the approval rate has risen, it has not returned to the pre-1962 level.

There are different ways of looking at the sharp drop in new drugs after the 1962 amendments tightening requirements for FDA approval. Not all the drop can be attributed to regulation. A backlog of scientific breakthroughs during the 1930s and 1940s had been depleted. The cost and difficulty of developing new useful products may have been rising, FDA or no FDA. Should we be dismayed by the decline in new drugs approved by the FDA? We have no reason to believe that the pre-1962 rate was the right rate. Nevertheless, the sharp rise in research and development and testing costs should induce pharmaceutical companies to concentrate their research in areas where both the discovery costs would be relatively low and the testing costs and testing time would be short. This means me-too drugs, not breakthroughs in areas not previously treatable, which might involve much longer and costlier testing before FDA approval. It takes ten to twelve years to develop a new pharmaceutical, and an estimated $231 million (half of this is the interest foregone by tying up capital for such a long time in R&D and testing).[33] The research process is full of uncertainty; a firm may test 4,000 substances to find five that merit human testing, only one of which will eventually be marketed.[34] With biotechnology, the uncertainties are different: a firm does not test numerous substances, it engineers new substances.

After 1972, the United States lost its lead in marketing new drugs and new breakthrough drugs.[35] Various changes in regulation have been designed to increase incentives to conduct research and cut the cost of developing new drugs. The reduced market life before the expiration of patents, a result of greatly increased time as well as cost of testing new drugs after 1962, a factor in the high price of new drugs, in 1986 led to the extension of the seventeen-year patent period to twenty-two years for some drugs whose review process by the FDA was exceptionally lengthy. But we are told that patents are irrelevant for the new genetic medicine because periods of development have been greatly shortened, and the effective market life has also been greatly reduced. I suspect that breakthrough technologies have a long market life, and many of those with a short market life perhaps should not have been approved at all, and it is just as well that their market life is short.

The testing process has been shortened for drugs possibly helpful for otherwise deadly diseases. In May 1987 the FDA ruled that victims of AIDS and other fatal diseases could buy experimental drugs. In October 1988 it provided for quick approval for breakthrough drugs; in both cases, it related concern for safety to the need, to the severity of the condition. Nevertheless, the prospect of liability litigation remains a deterrent to early introduction.

The incentives for FDA employees have been all in the direction of rejection; no one wants to be responsible for recommending approval of a new thalidomide. The external evaluators who lead separate careers, used in some other countries, can be more even-handed. Some new drugs are to be partly evaluated by outside contractors. The FDA will accept more studies conducted by other nations.

Undue stress on the goal of perfectly safe drugs has delayed and sometimes denied access to new drugs for people who had much to gain and often little to lose from using them. No system of tests can predict rare events very well, or effects that take long in showing up. Think of aspirin, how long it has been around, but new benefits and side effects have only recently been discovered. On the other hand, some counterweight is needed for the bias toward new drugs and procedures, both on the side of providers and of customers, which if unreined, increases the use of drugs and procedures too early in the learning curve. This is a very contentious issue; longer delays in getting a drug to market deprive some of the benefits of its use; on the other hand, more careful testing and evaluation spare others harmful side effects that might not have been detected otherwise. Since there is no dependable way to track most drugs once they are in the market, all the more need for some restraint. Reliance on voluntary reporting by individual physicians is a slow and unreliable way to learn.

A process of drug approval that is lengthy and costly raises prices because the firm's costs are higher, and because the period during which it can sell under patent protection is shorter. The desire for lower prices conflicts with the desire for safety, and since it implies lower profits, it also conflicts with the desire for more research and improved therapeutic products.

It is often claimed that there is much waste in pharmaceutical research, that competitive pressures drive firms to develop me-too drugs to obtain or retain market share. It is true that most research is directed at developing new chemical entities that differ only slightly from drugs already on the market. The claim that they are mere duplication, that they are developed only to compete with existing drugs, is overstated. Most of these me-too drugs are designed for improved efficacy or for a different range of efficacy, and/or for reduced side effects or for different side effects that render them more suitable than the existing drug for certain customers. Some simply displace their predecessors; others, because of advantages for some users (children, the elderly, individuals with particular dysfunctions) offer the physician a choice of medications that are equivalent but different. True, much of me-too drug development is wasteful; some of it is useless, some of it no improvement. It wastes not only research resources but production, advertising, and promotion funds. But if the FDA approves, there will be more of the same.

Extension of patent life to twenty-two years to make up for time consumed in FDA regulatory review also applies to medical devices, which have been regulated since 1976. The Center for Devices and Radiological Health, part of the FDA, will expedite review of products offering innovation versus copycats, and will differentiate simple low-risk products, which will get only an administrative review, from those requiring risk assessment. On the other hand, many tests and most procedures can be introduced without prior authorization. The only constraint on premature introduction, or introduction of procedures of questionable value, is the withholding of insurance coverage.

The prospect of coverage by Medicare, Medicaid, and private insurance companies is an important incentive for development of new drugs and procedures.[36] But insurance has biased innovation toward cost-increasing technology. The introduction of DRGs by Medicare should reduce this bias and should eventually reverse it as DRGs become the universal approach toward compensation.[37] Decisions on what new technology insurance should cover are critical influences on the choice of technology and in turn on R&D decisions. But the direction of influence is not entirely one-way; new technology leads to extension of insurance coverage.[38]

The major impact of third-party payments on the costs of new technology is to encourage its use and overuse by rendering physicians and their customers insensitive to costs. A secondary consequence is on the price of new technology. Since the customer is much less sensitive to price when he does not pay it directly than when he does, the supplier of new technology is likely to charge a higher initial price and to reduce it more slowly over time. The supplier's volume of sales is less dependent on price, and so is its market share once competitors arise.

Decisions on coverage can limit the overuse of technologies, new and old; can discourage their use in inappropriate ways or for inappropriate customers. What we have learned about excessive numbers of surgical procedures, overuse of tests and pharmaceuticals, suggests that limits on insurance coverage have not been used very effectively. Both physicians and their customers have a vested interest in more tests, more drugs, more procedures. And physicians are the ones who provide the information, who make a case for insurance coverage. Only in managed-care systems does insurance (prepayment) provide an effective means of limiting introduction of new technologies and overuse of technologies new and old. The DRG system should nudge hospitals in the direction of managed care. But both remain under countervailing pressure to acquire the latest technology, which, in hospitals, often must be overused to pay for itself. The conflict-of-interest problem of M.D. investment in pharmacies has largely disappeared (or shifted toward clinics and laboratories). There are reports of financial inducements by pharmaceutical firms to physicians to prescribe their expensive drugs, but no reason to believe that this is a major factor in their overuse. But hospitals profit (countering shortfalls elsewhere) by grossly overcharging for drugs given their customers.

Drugs are poorly covered by health insurance policies or Medicare. If they were to become more adequately covered, one could expect (1) higher prices for drugs; (2) a greater use of drugs; (3) an increased total amount spent on drugs; and (4) more R&D by pharmaceutical companies, especially on more new me-too drugs.

Technology and the Cost of Medical Care

What is the effect of new technology on the costs of medical care? This is a complex question. First, what is the rate of introduction of new technology? Is it increasing, decreasing, or neither? Second, what is the cost of new technology, and how rapidly does it fall as the technology ages? And third, how does the new technology affect the costs of treatment or the incidence of illness?

There is some evidence that the rate of development of new drugs has been declining, but such a trend cannot be extrapolated. Breakthroughs in basic science—molecular biology and genetics—and applications in genetic engineering and in reducing the trial-and-error element in new drug research accelerate the development of new drugs and promise to increase their number in the future.

We can distinguish between product and process innovation; product innovations open up new possibilities for treatment. Product innovations may be product adding or product substituting. Product-substituting innovations reduce medical risks or improve quality of existing treatment; their effect can raise or reduce costs, depending on their effectiveness. Product-adding innovations extend the reach of medical cure or treatment and are likely to increase costs. Halfway technologies are almost certain to raise costs. Pure process innovations cut the costs of doing what is already done. As indicated earlier, the present system of medical care and insurance biases innovation toward new products, toward halfway technologies, therefore toward higher costs. Health conditions for which there was no treatment become amenable to medical care; the scope for diagnosis and treatment is extended.

Some new technology offers treatment for medical conditions that formerly were untreatable; it expands the range of medical care. Organ transplants and a wide range of surgical procedures and prosthetic devices have been developed in recent decades, plus cures for pneumonia, tuberculosis, and other diseases formerly untreatable.

Other new technology improves the diagnosis and treatment of conditions that were already within the compass of medical care. In diagnosis we have advanced from X-rays to CT scanners and MRIs; in treatment, from aspirin to a wide spectrum of antibiotics. There are better treatments for bleeding ulcers, diabetes, epilepsy, and a wide range of infectious diseases. We cannot always quantify the improvements in reliability and precision of diagnosis, in quality of treatment or outcome. Even when we can apply some quantitative yardstick, such as bed days, or workdays lost, it is not equally applicable for all new technologies.

The new technology may be a cost-saving improvement over existing treatments (or diagnostic techniques). Improved outcomes may be obtained with no increase in costs or risks (or at reduced costs or risks). Finally, techniques may be developed that are not cost reducing, but outcome improving.

A new drug may cut short the duration of illness, reduce its severity, or reduce or eliminate hospital stays, thus cutting medical costs (e.g., penicillin). It may preclude the need for medical care (e.g., the polio vaccine), lowering costs. Or a drug suppressing the immune system may make possible tissue and organ transplants that could not have succeeded without it, thus raising medical costs. Lens replacements and laser surgery may save sight that could not have been saved in the past, again raising medical costs. But these are only the direct impacts of new technology. One should consider indirect impacts. Sight has been saved for many. There have been major gains in survival rates of victims of strokes and heart attacks. Such technical advances raise costs directly, by saving lives. They also raise costs indirectly because the individuals whose lives are saved live on to require additional medical care in the future. But this is an unacceptable position; it implies that we should all be stillborn. One has to weigh costs against benefits.

The best example of cost-reducing innovation is penicillin: it greatly reduced the capital and labor costs of treatment for a wide range of bacterial infections. It also improved outcomes: mortality rates fell, long-term impacts on health were reduced. Its net impact on health care was a reduction in costs. Another example is the development of vaccines for a number of childhood diseases, whose use involved much less cost than treatment of the cases that would have developed otherwise. One might claim that for some of the diseases prevented by vaccines there was no effective treatment (treatment was given nevertheless), and hence vaccines expanded the scope of medical care, not via treatment, but via effective prevention.

The assumption that previously untreatable conditions did not absorb health care resources may not be true. Sometimes caring costs more than curing because the process takes much longer. We have no treatment for influenza, but nevertheless examine, hospitalize; there is much expensive care, even if there is no cure. The same could have been said about pneumonia before the advent of antibiotics; we really had no treatment, but victims were hospitalized and incurred greater "medical" expenses when there was no cure than when a cure became available. Now that drug-resistant strains have evolved, expenses should rise again because treatments do not work and new strains may be more virulent. The cost of new technology is almost invariably higher than that of the old technology it displaces. CT scanners cost more than traditional X-rays. New technologies are more precise, more complex. The price of a new drug is high initially. The firm introducing a new drug has a temporary monopoly that permits it to charge a high price until its patent expires or until competitors develop substitute products. It needs to recover the up-front cost of research and development, testing and evaluation, including the costs of numerous failures, and to provide funds for developing other drugs. The seller does not know how much he will sell, or for how long, and must make conservative assumptions on market size, market share, and market life. The effect on health care costs depends not on price but on effectiveness: does it cure the illness promptly, avoiding much larger costs, or is it a palliative with little effect on other medical costs? The initial cost of penicillin was high, but it worked; aspirin was cheap, but it did not work.

New technology provides new opportunities for overtesting, overtreatment. Once a hospital has acquired expensive new equipment, it makes sense to use it as intensively as possible, to cover its costs. This intensive use does reduce the unit cost to the patient, but by greatly increasing the number of patients using the new technology. The availability of the new technology in one hospital places pressure on nearby hospitals to acquire the technology also; this proliferation makes it more difficult to spread costs by more intensive use, on the one hand keeping unit costs high as capacity is underutilized and on the other hand increasing the extent of overutilization of the new technology.

Increasing Costs of Research and Development

One reason for the rapidly rising costs of medical care is excessive competitive R&D, which results in too many therapeutically equivalent new products and in too much spending on advertising new products, all of which are encouraged by the availability of third-party payments. It is clear why, if cost is no object, many expensive new drugs, treatments, tests, and diagnostic procedures are used. The patent system obviously has something to do with excessive spending on R&D and the introduction of too many new drugs marginally superior to existing drugs, if superior at all. Competitors seek to develop a drug that will circumvent the market monopoly of a patented drug. Given the cost of doing this duplicative R&D, much less would be done if it were not possible to sell large amounts at high prices, that is, if there were no third-party payments. The competitive race results not only in duplication of new drugs but of new technology of all sorts. Other factors, which could not have been effective in the absence of third-party payments, are the not-so-subtle pressure by physicians for the latest drugs, and by patients also, in part the outcome of advertising campaigns by the manufacturers of medical products. In large cities there is too much duplication of expensive equipment and facilities; smaller cities have expensive equipment when they should use instead the equipment and facilities in larger cities nearby. If M.D.s and hospitals run by M.D.s were not prepared to compete in obtaining and using new technology, including drugs, manufacturers could not cover the costs of many of them and would have to reduce duplicative R&D. If hospitals and M.D.s could not recoup their costs, via a combination of overuse and higher charges, there would be less duplication of facilities and equipment, less overuse, and fuller capacity utilization.

But there are more fundamental forces behind rising costs. We can say that generally each new generation of technology costs a multiple of the preceding generation.[39] This is only partly an artifact of the normal high initial cost and declining cost with the passage of time: a comparison of X-rays that have been perfected and improved and produced by the tens of thousands with brand-new CT scanners turned out on a custom rather than assembly-line basis. The difference in initial cost of succeeding technological generations is also large, eventually so large that even with third-party payments, demand is constrained by cost and opportunities for economies of mass production are reduced or entirely eliminated. Costs of improvements as well as initial research and development costs must be spread over fewer and fewer units. The rising prices of new technology in turn compel health care organizations to make often excessive use of it as a means of spreading and recovering costs. To the extent that technological generations become shorter, as they may have been in recent decades, the effect of escalating original cost and shorter production runs is aggravated.

Costs tend to rise because the easy steps are taken first. Technical difficulty tends to increase exponentially. We can see this in the effort to establish the genetic basis of disease: those illnesses determined by a single gene were identified first; then those influenced but not determined by one or two genes; finally, and we are far from there yet, those whose genetic basis is much more complex—multiple genes, undeciphered relations among them in influencing the probability of disease. We see this in environmental research. Chlorination to destroy microorganisms in the water supply and pasteurization were simple. Identifying chemicals that cause cancers or a variety of noninfectious ailments from among a great number of prospects and isolating their influence from that of other causal agents is extraordinarily complicated. Producing vaccines that outwit the mutating variants of viruses and bacteria is not like devising the original smallpox vaccine. This is the basis of Nicholas Rescher's argument that technology faces diminishing returns.[40] If we compare the large amounts spent on research in recent years with the comparatively minuscule amounts spent in the 1930s and 1940s, which led to the sulfa drugs and antibiotics as well as to a number of valuable vaccines, one would have to agree. Yet the limitations of the steam engine were circumvented by the internal combustion engine and in turn by the jet engine. Each technological regime faces diminishing returns but is replaced by successors. It may just be that new technologies originally developed far from the health care industry—molecular genetics and computers and the arts of miniaturization—will give us a fresh start beyond the limits of the chemist and the scalpel.

There is another aspect to diminishing returns: the nature of the human species. We have come so far in the past two or three centuries, from an unhealthy life expectancy of less than thirty years to one that may soon approach eighty, much of it relatively free of sickness and debility, how much further is there to go?

Notes

1. Robert Kanigel,"Where Mind and Body Meet," *Mosaic* 17, no. 2 (Summer 1986): 52–60; Robert Ornstein and David Sobel, "Can the Brain Heal the Body?" *Washington Post,* May 3, 1987, B3; Jean Marx, "The Immune System 'Belongs in the Body,' "

Science 227 (March 8, 1985): 1190–92; Vernon Riley, "Psychoneuroendocrine Influences on Immunocompetence and Neoplasia," *Science* 212 (June 5, 1981): 1100–09.

2. Don Colburn, "Drug Prices: What's Up?" *Washington Post/Health,* December 15, 1992, 8–13, esp. 10.

3. Simon Rottenberg, "The Allocation of Biomedical Research," *American Economic Review* 57 (May 1967): 109–18.

4. Philip Abelson, "A View of Health Research and Care," *Science* 200 (May 28, 1978): 845.

5. Thomas Moore, *Lifespan* (New York: Simon and Schuster, 1993), 29–32, 237–39. See also S. Jay Olshansky, Bruce Carnes, and Christine Cassel, "In Search of Methusaleh: Estimating the Upper Limits to Human Longevity," *Science* 250 (November 2, 1990): 634–40. Since it is not possible to reduce infant mortality much more in absolute terms, or that of young and middle-aged adults, most further increase in life expectancy must come about through increasing the life span of those past sixty and particularly past seventy and eighty. This prospect should immediately raise the question of the quality of life extended.

6. Constance Holden, "Giving Mental Illness Its Research Due," *Science* 232 (May 30, 1986): 1084–85.

7. Ann Gibbons, "Exploring New Strategies to Fight Drug-Resistant Microbes," *Science* 257 (August 21, 1992): 1036–38.

8. George R. Siber, "Pneumococcal Disease: Prospects for a New Generation of Vaccines," *Science* 265 (September 2, 1994): 1385–87.

9. Jon Cohen, "Bumps on the Vaccine Road," *Science* 265 (September 2, 1994): 1371–73.

10. Raphael D. Dolin, "Antiviral Chemotherapy and Chemoprophylaxis," *Science* 227 (March 15, 1985): 1296–1303.

11. Jon Cohen, "Vaccines Get a New Twist," *Science* 264 (April 22, 1994): 503–5.

12. Barbara Culliton, "Emerging Viruses, Emerging Threat," *Science* 247 (January 19, 1990): 279–80.

13. Jon Cohen, "Childhood Vaccines: The R&D Factor," *Science* 259 (March 12, 1993): 1528–29.

14. Stanley Riddell, Kathe Watanabe, James Goodrich, et al., "Restoration of Viral Immunity in Immunodeficient Humans by the Adoptive Transfer of T Cell Clones," *Science* 257 (July 10, 1992): 238–40.

15. Antonio Lanzavecchia, "Identifying Strategies for Immune Intervention,"*Science* (May 14, 1992): 937–44.

16. Robert Plomin, Michael Owen, and Peter McGuffin, "The Genetic Basis of Complex Human Behavior," *Science* 264 (June 17, 1994): 1733–39. See also Eric S. Lander and Nicholas Schrok, "Genetic Dissection of Complex Traits," *Science* 265 (September 30, 1994): 2037–48; Jean Marx, "Dissecting the Complex Diseases," *Science* 247 (March 30, 1990): 1540–42.

17. Victoria Conti, "New Insights into Cancer, Psoriasis, and Other Major Health Problems," *NCCR Reporter,* March/April 1994, 4–11; Rick Weiss, "Scientists Making Gains against Inherited Diseases Find Their Task Harder Than Expected," *Washington Post/Health,* October 18, 1994, 12–15.

18. "Silver Thread, Thin Bones," *Science* 266 (October 21, 1994): 365.

19. Rachel Nowak, "Genetic Testing Set for Takeoff," *Science* 265 (July 22, 1994): 464–67; Peter T. Rowley, "Genetic Screening: Marvel or Menace?" *Science* 225 (July 13, 1984): 138–44.

20. W. French Anderson, "Human Gene Therapy," *Science* 256 (May 8, 1992): 808–13.

21. One might argue that bone-marrow transplantation, around for quite a few years, is a crude early form of genetic therapy. But it requires a compatible donor and suppression of the immune system. See Robertson Parkman, "The Application of Bone Marrow Transplantation to the Treatment of Genetic Diseases," *Science* 232 (June 13, 1986): 1373–78.

22. Weiss, "Scientists Making Gains against Inherited Diseases," 12–15.

23. Arno Motulsky, "Impact of Genetic Manipulation on Society and Medicine," *Science* 219 (January 14, 1983): 135–40; Leslie Roberts, "Ethical Questions Haunt New Genetic Technologies," *Science* 243 (March 3, 1989): 1134–36; Nelson Wivel and Leroy Walters, "Germ-line Gene Modification and Disease Prevention: Some Medical and Ethical Perspectives," *Science* 262 (October 22, 1992): 533–38.

24. C. Thomas Caskey, "Disease Diagnosis by Recombinant DNA Methods," *Science* 236 (June 5, 1987): 1223–29.

25. Leonard Scinto, Kirk Daffner, David Dressler, et al., "A Potential Noninvasive Neurobiological Test for Alzheimer's Disease," *Science* 266 (November 11, 1994): 1051–54.

26. Jacob Hanker and Beverly Giammara, "Biomaterials and Biomedical Devices," *Science* 242 (November 11, 1988): 885–92.

27. Stella Jones Fitzgibbons, "Making Artificial Organs Work," *Technology Review* 97, no. 8 (August/September 1994): 33–40.

28. Scott Veggeberg, "Probing the Brain," *NCRR Reporter* 18, no. 6 (November/December 1994): 12–13.

29. Marx, "Dissecting the Complex Diseases," 1540–42.

30. Henry Grabowski and John Vernon, "Consumer Protection Regulation in Ethical Drugs," *American Economic Review* 67 (February 1977): 359–64.

31. William S. Comanor, "The Political Economy of the Pharmaceutical Industry," *Journal of Economic Literature* 24 (September 1986): 1178–1217, esp. 1179.

32. Henry Grabowski, *Drug Regulation and Innovation* (Washington, D.C.: American Enterprise Institute, 1976).

33. Colburn, "Drug Prices: What's Up?" 8–13.

34. John Schwartz, "U.S. Drug-Testing Gantlet May Be World's Toughest," *Washington Post,* September 7, 1993, A9.

35. Mary Graham, "The Quiet Drug Revolution," *Atlantic Monthly,* January 1991, 34–40.

36. John Godderis, "Insurance and Incentives for Innovation in Medical Care," *Southern Economic Journal* (October 1984): 530–39.

37. Louis Garrison, Jr., and Gail Wilensky, "Cost Containment and Technology," *Health Affairs* 5 (Summer 1986): 46–58, esp. 50–51.

38. Burton Weisbrod, "The Health Care Quadrilemma: An Essay on Technological Change, Insurance, Quality of Care, and Cost Containment," *Journal of Economic Literature* 29 (June 1991): 523–52, esp. 524, 528.

39. Nicholas Rescher, *Unpopular Essays on Technological Progress* (Pittsburgh: University of Pittsburgh Press, 1980), 93–104.

40. Ibid., 99–103.

10

The Physician as Agent

Why discuss agency? In the days of the general practitioner with his little black bag, there was no need. But in an age of specialization, agency, or responsibility for the patient's welfare, is diffused. In the organized practice of medicine, hospitals in particular, but also in HMOs and other group practices, there are conflicts between the needs of patients and the demands of management. Imperfect agency is assumed in accounting for much over-supply of medical services.

What should the doctor do on behalf of the patient? Is some of the excess supply of services perhaps no more than a response to the excessive demands of patients or their underlying motivations? Is it appropriate? The literature on agency is of limited help. Much of it is concerned with how the principal should reward the agent so as to provide incentives to optimize the agent's behavior.[1] The relation between physicians and customers is different; the principal, or customer, has no say about prices or earnings, only about which primary-care doctor to see and whether or not to follow the M.D.'s recommendations. The customer's only options, if dissatisfied, are to seek another physician or institute a malpractice suit. And the customer often cannot judge, even after the fact, whether or not the M.D. has been a good agent in his behalf; the physician is the customer's main source of information. Nor, in most cases, is there professional consensus on a single standard of care.[2]

The burden of being a good agent for the customer falls mainly on the physician and the hospital. But in many cases the principal must also act as his or her own agent, assuming some responsibility for health-preserving or health-restoring behavior. The limits of agency in health services may be drawn by analogy with other kinds of insurance. The premiums on fire insurance for individuals depend on building materials, proximity to a fire hydrant, and the use of sprinkler systems and smoke detectors. Coverage does not apply in the case of arson by the policyholder. Life insurance premiums depend on age and sex. There may be lower premiums for lower-risk classes: smoking behavior and weight in relation to some norm. Coverage does not apply in the case of suicide. In the early days of air travel, air-travel-related deaths were not covered. By contrast, in health care the insurer cannot consider, and the agent cannot control, the patient's failure to seek medical treatment, the patient's failure or refusal to follow medical advice, or the patient's foolhardy pattern of behavior.

What Is Perfect Agency?

What is meant by perfect agency? Does the M.D. act as the patient would have acted had he or she had all the information available to the M.D.? Does the M.D. make the decisions, or at least the recommendations? Does the M.D. adopt the patient's risk-aversion behavior instead of making decisions as though he were a statistician? Does this imply that the M.D. will seek additional information via tests beyond the point where the additional expected benefit may be less than the expected costs and risks? Does the M.D. accommodate excess, unreasonable demand, which possibly poses greater risks than probable benefits?

There is a populist view that regards only passive representation as acceptable; it levels all differences, in this case the difference in knowledge of physician and customer. The physician must present as much information as possible to the customer about options, alternatives, and their pros and cons, then ask the customer to make the decision, knowing full well that the customer does not have all the knowledge, all the experience, available to the agent. The customer in turn is in no position to know whether all relevant options have been presented or whether they are based on correct diagnosis or whether their implications and probabilities are accurately reported. This alternative has very high costs for both parties. It bows to customer wishes, biases, not necessarily in the best interests of health. Fear of malpractice might be an inducement for the physician to place the burden of decision on the customer.

An older view of perfect agency sees the physician as responsible for the well-being of the customer, not as poll taker. When all procedures yield the same probable outcome, there are no ethical issues; the physician may also consider comfort, convenience, cost. The customer does not implicitly delegate benefit choices to the physician, only instrumental choices. Agency at one time implied that the physician would conduct an imaginary benefit-cost analysis, taking the financial circumstances of the customer and the family into account in recommending the amount, type, and quality of medical care. With third-party payments reducing the financial costs to near zero for most people, economic cost is no longer a concern (except insofar as third-party payers impose restrictions on reimbursement), and the physician becomes concerned solely with benefit and medical risk. Since the financial costs are only in part, often in small part, payments to the physician, he or she may not know what they are. The complete course of treatment for an individual often cannot be known in advance, and the known risks are statistical guidelines, whose relevance for a particular patient is uncertain. The cost still remaining is the harm that may be done by treatment, the risks of some diagnostic procedures, medication, surgery.

If all physicians share the same knowledge and the element of uncertainty is small, all should make the same recommendation. In fact they do not, and the question is to what extent they do not share the same knowledge, to what extent they react differently to the elements of risk and uncertainty associated with particular diagnostic procedures or treatments, and to what extent they do not act as proper agents in behalf of the customer and taint their recommendations with their own self-interest.

What should the physician do when the condition being treated is life-threatening and not self-terminating? Often the patient is not in a mental condition to express his views. There may be a living will, or the views of close relatives, or those of the patient when he or she was able to express them. A high-risk procedure may then be proper, if no other options promise a satisfactory outcome. One need not assume that under these conditions both principal and agent become risk prone. Risk is a relative, not an absolute, consideration. Russian roulette with only one empty chamber is a fail-safe procedure if the only alternative is all chambers loaded.

The customer's inevitable ignorance requires trust in the physician's decisions and recommendations, in the adequacy of the information provided when alternatives are left for the customer to select among. A relationship of trust applies mainly to physicians with whom one has long continuing contacts, primary-care physicians, a diminishing proportion of all physicians, engaged in diagnosis and in assessing the needs of specific individuals for treatment or referral. Contacts with specialists are infrequent, sporadic, often once only. Confidence here has to do with belief in technical ability, which cannot be based on long personal experience, only on information provided by others and on unreliable personal judgments. Primary-care doctors probably preserve much more of the traditional expected motivation of doctors than specialists. They retain more of the role of agent. The principal has the choice of primary-care doctors. Since they deal with a wide variety of patients, a wide variety of problems, it is very hard to compare their effectiveness even by other M.D.s, never mind by customers relying on others' subjective feelings, gossip.

It was easy for the physician to serve as the customer's agent half a century and more ago, when for most ailments there were few if any high-cost treatment options, when most of the costs of medical care were the physician's own fees, over which he or she had complete control. Now there are alternative treatment options, high-cost options where there were only low-cost options, and costs most of which are outside the individual physician's control. Instead of a single agent, the general practitioner, there is a proliferation of specialists and a shift of treatment from home and office to hospital settings where it is difficult to know who, if anyone, is the agent, where multiple agents' contribution to health outcomes may not be independent, none of whom have much information about the patient's attitudes and preferences.

The role of agency is inevitably delegated; the hospital or clinic has ultimate responsibility for the work of its employees performed on its premises, but hospitals are institutions, not individuals. Senior staff may supervise or monitor junior staff, doctors may monitor one another. The role of agency is split: the physician is an agent for the institution within which he or she works, an agent for other health care personnel, as well as ultimately for the patient. These roles often conflict.

Administrators are concerned not with any individual patient but with overall costs, revenues, decisions on investment in facilities. Physicians are interested in having the facilities they want to use and access to them. Staff physicians may be under some administrative control, but referring physicians are not. They pressure the administration to acquire capabilities, to improve quality, to improve access.[3]

Customers are better off in a hospital where the customer is king, a hospital whose main if not sole purpose is to heal the sick. Teaching hospitals face conflicting goals: teaching and research are the main concerns, with patients and their treatment a necessary input. We might interpret behavior in teaching hospitals as a response to social agency rather than private individual patient agency, but I'm doubtful.

Changes in legal doctrine have affected physician behavior. Informed consent emerged as definite legal doctrine only in the late 1950s. It increases defensive medicine and reduces innovation by the M.D.—two possible negative side effects of agency. Some court decisions have made the physician not only accountable for negligence but for the patient's physical condition, for acts of God. Such an inflated concept of the physician's responsibility also has negative consequences for customers; the M.D. is given an incentive to avoid treating high-risk patients or using high-risk procedures.[4]

The Right to Know

Legally, agency requires informed consent. Medical care may be one of the most secretive industries in society.

> Suspicious of price competition, susceptible to medical jargon, secretive in their evaluation of one another's work, reluctant to testify against one another in negligence proceedings, unwilling to criticize standard procedures in public, determined to keep notes and records so confidential that they remain inaccessible even to the patient . . . doctors . . . are themselves contributing causes of consumer ignorance. . . .[5]

We have laws on truth in lending, truth in labeling, truth in advertising, but many medical personnel seem to regard the withholding of information as their professional prerogative. Too many questions annoy them, and inquisitive customers are viewed simply as victims of anxiety. What are their motives, what the justifications, what should be done about it? Going from the highest to the basest of motives, first there is realization that information, even intentional misinformation, has therapeutic value. The mental and emotional attitude of the patient is important; if nothing else, it affects the willingness and ability of the customer to follow a prescribed course of treatment. A physician may overstate the seriousness of a condition, minimize risks of treatment, or overstress the likely consequences of continuing in accustomed ways, as a means of motivating the patient toward the best course of action. Even where attitude cannot influence outcomes, where death is certain, there may be no purpose in dire predictions. Let the patient enjoy what life remains with some false hope. Sometimes it is a question of giving a customer time to adjust to a permanent disability. Or the next of kin are informed, the patient is not (or at times, vice versa, but then it is the customer's decision, not the doctor's). These considerations assume that the physician has deep understanding of the mentality of the customer, understanding often lacking in this age of specialization.

But in fact concern for the customer often has little to do with the withholding of information. The busy physician wants to move customers along and not use up time to explain; the physician does not know, or is unsure, and does not wish to tarnish an image of infallibility; test results are inconclusive, or lab reports may be unreliable; the physician does not really feel that the customer has the right to know or fears a loss of control once the customer becomes too knowledgeable to follow the physician's decisions blindly. Or the physician hates to be the harbinger of bad news, although that is an important part of medical work.[6]

I suspect that the value of the physician's time is the main nonaltruistic factor limiting disclosure of information. That other factors are important is suggested by the limited use physicians make of leaflets on illnesses, which could deal with a high proportion of the medical conditions on which patients are poorly informed and might be pardonably curious about, and which would save much time spent in repetitive explanations. Another example is the resistance of physicians to the sale of the *Physicians' Desk Reference* to nonphysicians—a battle long since lost—and the absence of copies from any doctor's waiting room I have ever visited. (I am not aware of any effort to bar the use of computer software programs such as Medline, which make it easy for anyone to locate summaries of recent technical articles on every condition and procedure. It would be impossible.) Why are physicians so reluctant to permit access to information on contraindications for particular pharmaceuticals, on their side effects? One explanation is that general availability might considerably reduce the amount of medication taken; it might convert large numbers into practicing Christian Scientists, perhaps reduce the frequency of doctors' visits; another is that it would certainly reduce the passive compliance of customers; they would ask too many questions.

Medical personnel are reluctant to acknowledge customers' rights of access to their medical records. (These rights have legal status in some states, not in others.) Probably time cost is the major factor; access will lead to many questions. Access makes patient contact less pleasant; the patient is more troublesome; the patient who asks questions may also question the decisions of medical personnel, and too much information may increase the chances of legal actions against them. The customer may choose to delegate all decisions to the physician without seeking information. But it should be a choice made consciously, not forced by the customer's ignorance of rights to information.

The role of agent for the customer is not compatible with provision of information only on a "need to know" basis, with withholding information requested by the customer. It is true that full information is out of the question; few customers would have the background to understand it. Truth in drug labeling, truth in diagnosis, can never take the quantifiable form of, or attain the precision of, a statement on the annual yield of a note or the weight of the contents of a can. Truth in medical care calls for probability statements. In fact, many M.D.s do not know; often no one knows. Adequate statistical information on the outcome of some procedures has not been collected, and statistical information is of questionable relevance with specific individuals. Less ignorance could lead to a more optimal demand for medical care.

So far we have considered the customer's right to know only about his or her own status and prospects and the physician's responsibilities and dilemmas in the same context. What about the right to know about the qualifications of physicians, hospitals, and other health delivery institutions so that the individual may have some basis for choosing among them? If this involves agency, it is from an industry and institutional perspective, a collective agency responsibility on the one hand and a right on the other. The industry has always regarded comparisons as odious and resisted advertising as unethical, although they are the essence of competitive behavior, consumer choice, and quality control in other industries. True, comparisons of hospitals in terms of mortality rates are invalid because case mixes differ. The same is true of physicians; there are problems with performance ratings. It is much easier to compare specialists in cardiac surgery than general surgeons; easier to compare general surgeons than internists, because of the greater diversity of practice of the latter, the greater difficulty in judging outcomes. The best specialists, those who may handle the most troublesome cases, could show up badly.

Cost comparisons also need to be made with extreme care. But in many cases valid comparisons are possible. We know that hospitals with over 200 cardiac surgical procedures a year have lower mortality rates than hospitals with a much smaller number of procedures. We know that some physicians have a disproportionate number of malpractice suits brought against them compared with others in the same specialty. This may not be a reasonable indicator of quality of care, but the number of cardiac surgical procedures is. Blue Cross–Blue Shield and other insurance companies have information on differences in quality and in cost of care that is not made available to their policyholders.

What about the general practitioner, the internist, as a source of information for his customers about hospitals and specialists? This responsibility falls clearly within a strict concept of agency. Hospital referrals are almost always the hospital in which the physician has staff privileges, the hospital that is most conveniently located from the physician's standpoint. A choice of physicians is almost invariably an implicit choice of hospitals as well. Most general practitioners have an old-boy network of specialists to whom they refer their customers. A choice of general practitioners is then also an implicit choice of the set of specialists and the hospitals to which the specialists refer. The customer is not offered a choice, nor the information on the basis of which to make an informed choice. Conversely, the choice of hospital, if that were made by a customer, would be an implicit choice of specialists as well. Some relaxation of physician staff privileges would lead to more unbiased recommendations, more information. Do physicians send their families, and themselves, to the same hospitals, the same specialists, to which they refer their customers? This is the litmus test.

The solution of one problem usually leads to a different problem, and the above instances of imperfect agency are no exception. If all customers had complete and unbiased information on the best hospitals and the best specialists for whatever ails them, the result would be a severe rationing problem: which patients get the best treatment, which must do with second-best? Not everyone can have the best general practitioners or specialists, even if there were consensus on who they are. For the best would be overbooked, others might be underworked. This is a fundamental difference between the demand for medical services and the demand for most goods. In the long run there is no limit on the number of Cadillacs or Chevrolets produced; it is relative price that sorts out buyers of one or the other. Third-party payments greatly weaken the influence of relative price in health care, but even if there were no third-party payments, not everyone, even not everyone who can afford it, can go to the Mayo Clinic. The American public opposes rationing, but rationing in the health care field is unavoidable. This fact makes proper agency in referrals difficult to assess.

Ethical Issues

So far, agency has been discussed in terms of testing, diagnosis, treatment of disease. Not all ailments can be treated. Testing and diagnosis may reveal the presence of conditions unsuspected by the customer because they caused no symptoms at the time. What are the implications of agency in providing information? Does the patient wish to know about conditions which, until known, cause no discomfort or concern? Certainly a patient, once he is informed, will be concerned. Does the patient wish to have the ailment labeled, even though there is no treatment? Should the customer's wishes be determining, or is there a higher ethic to guide the physician? Even if the patient wishes to know, there is the possibility that once being informed, the patient wishes he or she had not found out. For by definition the desire to know in this context is based on ignorance of what is to be learned. In fact the patient may really wish to be reassured, to be told that he or she does not suffer from a dread disease, that whatever the condition, it can be alleviated or eliminated. Often the news is bad. Does the desire to know extend to bad news? Even if it does, the physician may be in a position to judge the consequences of information for the patient, which are in many cases themselves harmful. More information is not necessarily better than less. And the physician may then regard his or her role as agent to include both knowing what there is to tell, deciding what the customer wishes to know, and judging the reaction of the customer, and of the customer's environment, to the knowledge once irrevocably imparted.

If the condition can be treated, then by all means agency requires that the patient be told, insofar as knowing is a condition for following the recommended treatment. On the other hand, if nothing can be done, it is not clear that information is better than concealment. If the customer may die at any time from the rupture of an inoperable aneurysm deep within the brain, is there any purpose in saying so? Is there any purpose in telling some member of the family? This is ultimately situation ethics. All may be spared anxiety by being kept in ignorance. But perhaps steps should be taken by the customer, or by some member of the family, in anticipation of sudden death: a will, insurance, other precautions. It is a matter of judgment: is death likely soon, or is it an increased probability that may not eventuate for many years? We are all, in Lenin's words, dead men on furlough, and the knowledge that one has a shorter statistical life expectancy than another should not per se be cause for concern. It is also a question of how long the information may be kept from the individual at risk. An aneurysm may be revealed only by death; an incurable cancer, on the other hand, eventually reveals itself, voiding the precautions of the physician.

Perhaps the most difficult issues arise out of the discovery of serious genetic defects. If the defect implies that the individual will at some future time develop an untreatable condition, there is no difference from eventual catastrophes not of genetic origin; there may be no purpose in informing the patient, and the patient would probably not wish to know. If the defect means that the patient is in a higher-risk class, but certain precautionary steps, diet for individuals prone to diabetes for instance, may significantly reduce the risk, then the benefits of information clearly outweigh any other considerations. But the information may also refer to the probability of genetically defective offspring. Prospective parents may wish to know and have a right to know the prospects for their children. If the prospective parents are prepared to cancel a genetic error by abortion, should the fetus have Down's syndrome for instance, then even a high probability of severe genetic defects can be accepted; the parents must be informed in advance. If parents are not willing to accept an abortion, then it is not clear that information provided by amniocentesis fulfills any useful function; only information prior to conception has any bearing on parental decisions. They may choose to avoid pregnancy if the probability of a genetic defect is high.

Another dilemma of agency refers to the technological imperative, or prestige and research goals. There was a day, before the wide availability of third-party payments and sensitivity to civil rights, when M.D.s used charity patients for experimental purposes. The use may not have been more than withdrawal of a few cc. of blood, but it was done under the guise of diagnosis and treatment, without informing the patients (truly patients, not customers). This supply has nearly disappeared. But the practice has not. Overuse of new technological instruments, which involves improper use of agency, is widespread, often but not always under pressure from hospitals, which need to pay for them. Interns need experience. Experimental treatment for dying patients is often justified, but the true motivation may be hidden.

One can understand why some cancer patients seek laetrile treatments and why the M.D. must deny them—there is no evidence that they help, and they do harm if they preempt alternative treatments that might prove effective. But why should the terminal cancer victim submit to, in fact demand, injection with poisons, radiation, which makes him horribly sick, which make his dying a ghastly suffering? But some do, and how should their agent respond? Refuse? If they were nobly subjecting themselves to experimental treatment in the hope that their manner of dying would add one cubit to our knowledge of cancer, might benefit some who survive them, we might regard them as saints and heroes. The doctors who treat them may well regard them as no longer fit for any human purpose save that of experimental animals. But the patients, or victims, or their families, rarely are so self-sacrificing and other-considerate. Their motivation is almost invariably fear of dying, reluctance to accept the inevitable. It is not hope but fear that drives them to such depths.

Malpractice as Imperfect Agency

The view now prevails that medical care is not a service like any other, access to which and the quality of which depend on individual ability and willingness to pay. On the contrary, every individual is believed to have a right to the best or at least to high-quality medical care in practically unlimited amounts. This attitude could not have come to prevail under a fee-for-service system of medical care; it is one outcome of the dominance of third-party payments. The fact that patients pay only a small fraction of the cost makes them more demanding of both quality and quantity. The explosion in the number of malpractice suits, in the size of the awards, and in the costs of malpractice insurance are in part the consequence of nearly free medical care. There are other causes, such as changes in legal doctrine, increased numbers of high-risk procedures, perhaps the surplus of lawyers, and a reduced acceptance and respect for medical personnel and services (the latter may itself reflect the fact that their services are nearly free).

Malpractice suits may be regarded as a result of breach of implicit agency contracts, as attempts by the patient to enforce such contracts, and/or to collect damages resulting from breach of contract. The prevalence of third-party payments, with insurers determining what procedures are reimbursable and at what rates, means that some decision-making power has been delegated by the patient to the insurer. The insurer and the physicians are both agents of the customer, but with conflicting interests.[7]

Malpractice suits have more to do with relationships than with procedures. Their proliferation is a consequence of the breakdown of an agency relationship as a result of specialization and the shift of care to hospital settings with multiple agents. The customer usually cannot judge the quality of the agent's performance or his or her compliance with the principal's wishes. In solo practice, often no one can, short of malpractice litigation that investigates performance. (If customers could distinguish quality, a few M.D.s would be vastly overbooked, many would be semiunemployed.) But in hospitals, HMOs, group practices, physicians can assess each others' performance and take measures to discipline the incompetent and the negligent and to correct their mistakes. They can act as agents once removed in behalf of the customer. The fact that in many cases they have been reluctant or unwilling to impose restrictions on fellow physicians gravely at fault is another reason for the explosion of malpractice suits and costs.[8] In hierarchies (hospitals, HMOs) the physician is agent and principal simultaneously. There is a tendency for physicians to see themselves as agents of the institution in which they work, and of their profession, sometimes in conflict with their role as agents once removed of the customer at risk.

The suggestion that the threat of malpractice claims contributes toward perfect agency rests on several assumptions. The first is that all malpractice suits are sincere, none malicious or merely profiteering from legal opportunities and insurance coverage. This is not entirely correct. The more frequent resort to countersuits should reduce the number of frivolous charges of malpractice. The second is that the physician has perfect insurance options. In fact this is not the case. His policy may not be renewed, or rates may be increased, as a result of adverse judgments or even too many suits. If these possibilities that modify his behavior toward avoidance of malpractice claims did not exist, the physician might be subject to "moral hazard," a cavalier attitude toward the risk of malpractice because of the fact of insurance coverage. Either zero risk of malpractice claims or perfect insurance would lead the physician to behave differently from his patients in regard to risk and uncertainty. The third assumption is that the physician's attitude toward risk and uncertainty with respect to malpractice claims and termination of insurance coverage is the same as his or her attitude toward diagnosis and treatment of customers. This is patently not true, since in malpractice litigation the physician stands to lose possibly very large sums and even the right to practice medicine (i.e., to future income). This is more like the patient's reaction to the possible loss of life and limb than to an objective calculation of costs and benefits in terms of their statistical probability of net benefit.

Proliferation of malpractice suits and of large awards is not a healthy development. That the customer should have legal recourse in cases of incompetent or negligent treatment is beyond question. But certainly doctors have not suddenly become less competent and more negligent and more damaging. Many patients are disillusioned, not because of M.D. malfeasance or nonfeasance, but because they expected the improbable. The status of medical practice as a scientific endeavor, of medical knowledge as omnicompetent, has been oversold to a population only too prone to expect and believe in simplistic mechanical or chemical solutions to complex and often insoluble problems. We believe that all problems have solutions, and if they are health problems, then M.D.s must have the solution. Therefore the customer has a right, not to good health care, but to good health. To some extent M.D.s have aggravated the problem by not being open and frank with their patients, fearing to destroy the patients' faith in some cases, wishing to minimize anxiety, or demands, hassle on the part of the patients in many cases, in some cases to reinforce the image in which they bask, although every physician knows enough about the limits of the healing art to avoid that temptation. As long as competent physicians exercise the care that is reasonable under the circumstances, the profession and the industry should not be held accountable for undesired consequences. Our understanding of many medical areas lacks a scientific base. Furthermore, customers are different, so neither a deep scientific understanding nor previous experience with other customers can serve as perfect guides for individual therapy. The development of treatments for medical conditions previously considered untreatable will increase the number of patients suffering adverse effects. The frequency of iatrogenic disease is often cited as an indictment of medical care, whereas to some extent it is an indicator of the extent of good medical care as well.

Is overtesting, overtreatment, and the practice of defensive medicine in response to the abstract threat of malpractice suits in fact perfect agency? Is it a response to the explicit or implicit demands of the customer? A patient's right to overtesting, overtreatment is analogous to the right to have a fire station next door, or to have the loss of assets by fire, or of life and limb, assessed and compensated at the loser's (or his or her dependents') subjective valuation, rather than on the basis of a market value or disinterested objective assessment. The hypothesis here is that the customer is more risk averse than the physician; that the customer's subjective odds are more conservative than the statistical odds that might guide the physician; that hence the customer overestimates the potential benefits and underestimates the potential costs (including possible adverse side effects). The physician is coerced by the threat of malpractice into behaving as if he accepted the patient's attitude toward risk and uncertainty.

The generalization of malpractice claims from physicians and their organizations to pharmaceutical companies and their products is a particularly dangerous development because it slows the introduction of new drugs, may adversely affect pharmaceutical research, causes the withdrawal of some drugs that are helpful or even essential for some individuals, and is threatening our supply of some vaccines as pharmaceutical companies discontinue production, deciding that the potential profits are not worth the legal costs and potential penalties, and certainly not worth the bad publicity. Almost any drug will cause adverse reactions in some patients, even when prescribed and taken according to sound medical practice. To be fair, these should be balanced against the effects they would have experienced in the absence of treatment, which are not counted as iatrogenic disease.

There must be some limit on liability, not only for doctors and hospitals, but also for producers of pharmaceuticals and health care equipment and supplies. Ceilings on individual awards in malpractice cases are being imposed by state after state. Some would restrict the use of contingency fees, but that could price poor claimants out of the malpractice market, and it is not clear that contingency fees persuade many lawyers to pursue dubious cases. The evidence is not that there are too many malpractice suits, but not enough, that most cases of negligence resulting in harm to the patient never result in any adversarial proceedings or penalties of any kind. From this standpoint, malpractice is a second-best approach, given the failure of the medical profession to police itself adequately.[9]

The role of the pharmaceutical company as agent is clearly different from that of the physician. It is at arm's length, to unknown users of its products, largely intermediated by physicians, although the information accompanying each container of drugs goes directly to the user. There are cases of misinformation via failure to inform physicians, users, and even the FDA of harmful side effects observed during trials that should be taken into account in approving and prescribing. This is a violation of basic agency. FDA approval should exempt manufacturers from claims not based on faulty manufacturing, packaging, storage, or information. Any such exemption should be accompanied by an improved process for periodic FDA review, as new evidence accumulates that might qualify the initial approval. Present possibilities for almost indefinite extension of the statute of limitations on product liability claims need to be constrained, for they amount to a sword of Damocles that magnifies insurance costs and threatens supply.

Is Private Agency Possible? Socially Desirable?

Is perfect agency always socially desirable? What is perfect agency from the viewpoint of the patient is overtesting, overtreatment from the standpoint of society, assuming that the M.D. seeks to be a perfect agent by adopting the patient's preferences.

There are a priori reasons to expect that the M.D. will not seek to be a perfect agent. Departures from perfect agency depend largely on the method of compensation. An M.D. compensated on a fee-for-service basis has an incentive to overtest, overtreat, to take a more serious attitude toward every illness than is warranted by the facts. Excessive surgery is the extreme case of agency failure (although method of compensation is not the only factor inducing unnecessary surgery). In the case of third-party payment, there is implicit collusion between principal and agent in favor of excessive services and often in favor of high-tech, high-risk treatments. Perfect agency in this case may be socially undesirable. When the patient pays, which was the traditional situation, there is implicit conflict between the physician's desire for income, or wish to submit to the technological imperative, and the limited means of the patient. The outcome of perfect agency in this case may also be socially undesirable. Payment on a salary basis, unrelated to the number of visits, to the number of procedures a physician performs, leads to the possibility of an opposite bias: undertesting, undertreatment, a casual attitude toward illness. So does capitation, or a fixed payment per patient for a given diagnosis. This is a universal problem. In many jobs and occupations there is some measure of individual performance, and pay may be linked thereto. But, in most, no easy measure is available, and as with the physician, we rely on "professionalism," on what Thorstein Veblen called the "instinct of workmanship."

Two considerations modify the effect of compensation on behavior. One is the physician's workload and attitude toward leisure. The other is what is widely labeled "professional ethics." If the M.D. has a strong preference for leisure, which tends to be greater the longer the workweek happens to be, he or she will tend to undertest and undertreat. The M.D. will also be biased toward the procedures that economize on time: hospitalization rather than office visits, tests and prescriptions rather than examinations, referrals to specialists rather than primary-care treatment. This tendency is reinforced if compensation is on a salary basis; it is counterbalanced somewhat if compensation is on a fee-for-service basis. Agency is involved, assuming that quality of care is affected by these decisions.

The supply of M.D.s will also affect agency. In times of a surplus, the typical M.D. will have a bias toward more services, more aggressive treatment, since he or she is short on income and long on time. During a shortage, the M.D. is short on time and perfect agency may mean sacrifice of leisure. For perfect agency, the supply of M.D.s should be large enough that their demand for leisure does not interfere with their acting as perfect agents; but then there may be an unsatisfied desire for additional income, which would interfere. Decisions of primary-care physicians to refer or not to refer to a specialist may be affected by their demand for leisure in the former case, for income in the latter.

As already mentioned, the technological imperative and the ethical desire to cure introduces a bias on the side of the physician and often on the side of the customer toward the latest, often experimental, tests, treatments, procedures. Perfect agency in this case may be considered socially undesirable.

Professional ethics would rule out all these considerations: amount or form of compensation, time availability, technological biases. But they cannot be ignored; if the physician is short on time, overburdened with patients, it becomes impossible to be a perfect agent; in other cases it is possible, but not always desirable. No system of compensation, no supply of M.D.s, assures perfect agency. Ultimately there is no substitute for professional ethics. Peer review, which is the main way of overseeing professional ethics, has two limitations. The first is the normal hazard of the old-boy network, the mutual protection society. How can peer review guarantee exposure, correction, prevention of "unethical" or professionally substandard behavior? The second (and it is not a criticism) is that peer review can only enforce technical standards; it is not guided, nor can it be, by patient preferences. Nor does it normally consider social costs and benefits. There is no reason why peer review could not be modified to consider social costs and benefits; in fact, technical judgment is ultimately unanchored, meaningless without such considerations. (Should there be heart transplants and who should get them precede judgments concerning the competence of a transplant operation.) But there is no way a peer review can consider the preferences of individual patients. The question is whether these preferences, if at odds with considerations of social welfare, should be weighed at all.

The physician and the health care delivery organization are under conflicting pressures from patients and their agents on the one hand, from governments and other third-party payers on the other. Patients pressure M.D.s under the threat of malpractice suits (and, as a doctor surplus grows, under the threat of changing doctors) to use all tests, to try all treatments. Defensive medicine and overdoctoring (and malpractice insurance) inevitably raise the costs of medical care. Absurdly large awards in malpractice suits drive defensive practice, raise medical costs for the rest of us, in premiums and taxes if in no other way (something victims of malpractice have no right to do, even if their cause is just, and many suits reflect neither physician carelessness nor incompetence, but opportunity, greed, an unreasonable expectation of favorable outcomes, or a free-floating desire for vengeance). Ceilings on awards are necessary not just to protect physicians' right to practice but to spare the rest of us the resulting high prices, premiums, taxes. The concept of agency cannot be stretched to require an obstetrician to practice the specialty in a state where the insurance premium is not much less than the doctor's probable income from delivering babies. There are ways of punishing the negligent doctor, of protecting the public, without punishing everyone else: restrictions or temporary or permanent revocation of the license to practice (something almost never done), required training and retraining. Let the physician who is at fault, rather than all physicians, and all patients, pay.

In the absence of third-party payments it would not be possible for physicians to increase their fees and services sufficiently to afford malpractice insurance. Although some overtesting and overtreatment is genuine defensive medicine, some of it is nothing but greed given a credible cover.

Who shall be my agent's keeper? In a system where the patient confronts not a single general practitioner but a whole battery of specialists, there is more information, more opportunity for generating information about proper care. It is more difficult for ignorance, incompetence, irresponsibility, or plain human error to escape detection. Doctors are the ones, often the only ones, to determine whether or not one of their own is at fault. But too many doctors are like the famous monkeys; they see no evil, hear no evil, speak no evil. They fall short in the agency task of disciplining one another, reducing or avoiding the occasion for further breach of agency.[10] One might say that malpractice litigation and malpractice insurance are largely the by-products of this collective failure of the fraternity. As improvements are made in state after state in disciplining errant members of the profession, in some cases removing their license to practice, one might hope that the number of suits, the amounts recovered, the premiums for malpractice would all go down.

Notes

1. David Sappington, "Incentives in Principal-Agent Relationships," *Journal of Economic Perspectives* 5, no. 2 (Spring 1991): 45–66. See also Bengt Holmstrom, "Moral Hazard in Teams," *Bell Journal of Economics* 13 (Autumn 1982): 324–40.

2. Gavin Mooney and Mandy Ryan, "Agency in Health Care: Getting beyond First Principles," *Journal of Health Economics* 12 (July 1993): 125–35.

3. Richard Epstein, "Medical Malpractice: Its Cause and Cure," in *The Economics of Medical Malpractice,* ed. Simon Rottenberg, 245–67, esp. 248, 265 (Washington, D.C.: American Enterprise Institute for Public Policy Research, 1978).

4. Jeffrey Harris, "The Internal Organization of Hospitals: Some Economic Implications," *Bell Journal of Economics* 8 (Fall 1977): 467–82. Informed consent may require a medical education and a good understanding of statistics, and if it does, there must be wide scope for the independent judgment of competent M.D.s, including the right to make mistakes. Doctors do not have the right to refuse treatment to patients who may not respond well to standard treatment; in fact, they may not be able to identify them in advance. Hence one may argue that the doctor is denied the right of informed consent in choosing patients.

5. David Reisman, *Market and Health* (New York: St. Martin's Press, 1993), chaps. 2, 3; see esp. 17.

6. Bowen Hosford, *Making Your Medical Decisions* (New York: Frederick Ungar, 1982), chap. 9.

7. Åke Blomqvist, "The Doctor as Double Agent: Information Asymmetry, Health Insurance and Medical Care," *Journal of Health Economics* 10 (May 1991): 411–32.

8. Susan Schmidt, "Doctors Rarely Lose Licenses," *Washington Post,* January 10, 1988, A1, 16–17.

9. Susan Schmidt, "Panel Has Difficulty Determining Incompetence," *Washington Post,* January 11, 1988, A1, 6–7.

10. William Goode, "The Protection of the Inept," *American Sociological Review* 32 (February 1967): 5–19, esp. 7.

11

Prevention: Environmental and Behavioral Modification

Before the Industrial Revolution, the average life expectancy was in the twenties; the preindustrial environment was deadly. Industrial civilization, although it has created new risks, has attained life expectancy in the upper seventies. Health and life have been improved in three ways: by altering the environment to reduce its threats; by protecting individuals and populations from environmental threats; and by learning to treat illness and injury.

In some instances, there are tradeoffs: prevention versus protection versus treatment. In other cases, we have no choice: we lack treatment for most viruses, but we can vaccinate or quarantine; we cannot protect individuals from polluted outdoor air, but we can reduce pollution. How do we allocate resources between public health prevention (environment), individual prevention (behavior), and treatment? Is prevention just an added cost of health care, or is it a means of reducing medical care needs and spending?

If we measure the conquest of disease in terms of mortality and life expectancy, the first great step forward was the dramatic fall in infant and child mortality in the late nineteenth and early twentieth centuries, almost entirely the result of improvements in prevention via public health measures: safe drinking water, sewage disposal, reduction in disease vectors. The second great advance, in the first half of the twentieth century, was a combination of prevention and treatment: new vaccines, further improvements in public health, food inspection, culminating in the antibiotic revolution of the 1940s. The third advance, in which we find ourselves, is defensive as well as preventive: staving off, slowing down the killers of middle and old age, prolonging the lives of the elderly instead of saving the lives of the young. It involves new medical technology, modification of lifestyles, and new measures for environmental modification, in particular the elimination or reduction of harmful chemicals rather than microorganisms.

Table 11.1

Trends in Infant Mortality and Life Expectancy

Year	Infant Mortality (per thousand births)	Life Expectancy
1900–1904	141.4	47.3 (1900)
1910–1914	116.7	50.0 (1910)
1920	85.8	54.1
1930	64.6	59.7
1940	47.0	62.9
1950	29.2	68.2
1960	21.6	69.7
1970	16.8	70.8
1980	12.6	73.7
1990	9.2	75.4
1992	8.5	75.7

Source: U.S. Bureau of the Census, *Statistical Abstract of the United States* (Washington, D.C.: Government Printing Office, various years).

The Old Prevention and the New

Most of the gain in life expectancy this century has nothing to do with medical care and a great deal to do with preventive measures adopted or more widely practiced in the first half of the century. Maintenance of these measures is essential to preserve most of the gains we have achieved. Life expectancy increased by 20.9 years in the first half of the century, only 7.2 years in the next forty. The large increase in life expectancy, 5.3 years, in the first decade of antibiotics, the 1940s, was almost as large as in the next forty years, a period that witnessed a doubling of the ratio of physicians to population (Table 11.1).

The important preventive measures of the past include chlorination of water supplies, sewage disposal, vaccination against infectious diseases, pasteurization of milk, inspection of food supplies, requirements for reporting certain diseases, procedures for quarantining victims of specified diseases, and the elimination of disease vectors: mosquitoes, flies, rats, and fleas.

The earliest stage of prevention was based, as was much medicine at the time, on the "germ" theory of disease (although concern with water quality and sewage disposal preceded it). It involved two approaches. The first was the elimination of microbes and their hosts, which might serve as disease vectors. The second stage aimed at protecting individuals by creating resistance or immunity to particular microbes, primarily through vaccination. If enough people are protected, it is possible to eliminate the disease in some cases, such as smallpox; in other cases, where animal hosts exist, elimination may not be possible. Most of the potential of this approach has been attained in advanced countries, and even in most developing nations, resulting in population explosions through sharp declines in mortality, particularly infant and child mortality.

Vaccination needs reemphasis. Too many preschool children have not been vaccinated, and measles epidemics, among others, have reappeared. New vaccines have been developed for diseases for which we have no effective treatment, and new vaccines have become necessary for illnesses that formerly could have been treated effectively with antibiotics. The development of resistance to most antibiotics by some strains of pneumococcus means that the elderly should be vaccinated. As the frequency of infection by diseases for which we have vaccines declines, the value of the vaccine as a preventive also declines. There is a dilemma: when an illness becomes very rare, the risks of vaccination can exceed the risks of catching it. But if people are not vaccinated, the disease comes back, eventually in epidemic numbers.

The third stage, in the midst of which we find ourselves (and so does medicine) has moved beyond the germ theory; it is based on "environmental" and "lifestyle" theories of disease. The main thrust of recent legislation has been aimed at reducing environmental threats: reduction of health-threatening sources of air and water pollution and a variety of measures to reduce health hazards in the workplace and in places of residence: poisons, carcinogens, allergens. The Environmental Protection Agency (EPA) and the Occupational Safety and Health Administration (OSHA) and the Consumer Products Safety Commission are new agencies of public health. The Food and Drug Administration (FDA) is an older instrument. A fourth stage, the "genetic" theory of disease, although by no means new, is only now developing the scientific base for public health policies (genetic testing) and preventive medical treatment. These stages do not supplant one another; they supplement.

The Ecological Approach

Rene Dubos noted that the incidence of a wide range of diseases was related to social conditions; social upheavals and the early stages of the Industrial Revolution, displacing millions from their accustomed life, urbanizing a rural population, rapidly changing adaptive requirements, led to a rise in the incidence of disease.[1] Harvey Brenner showed that when economic conditions are good and improving, society at peace, the outlook optimistic, there is less illness and injury. Deteriorating economic circumstances and social conflict are associated with higher rates of many illnesses and injuries.[2] An increasing disparity in mortality between socioeconomic groups has been noted in this country and in the United Kingdom, despite equalization of access to medical care.[3] It may be more than coincidence that the number of days of restricted activity per capita was substantially higher in 1980 (19.1), a recession year, than it was in 1970 (14.6), but declined during the prosperous 1980s, rising again in the early 1990s, a period of recession. The number of days of bed disability exhibited the same pattern.[4]

Health as an interaction of environment and behavior, which might be called an ecological approach, is a traditional view that now is better founded on facts and disposes of technological resources. It believes that much disease can be prevented by individual and/or group efforts, that much disease has to do with the way we live and how we cope with the problems of life. Long institutionalized through the Public Health Service, recently this view has been conquering new territory, via EPA and OSHA. The surgeon general's warning against tobacco opened up a new front, which former Surgeon General C. Everett Koop is trying to extend to obesity. In fact there are two strategies, internal to the individual or behavioral, and external or environmental, which are radically opposed in the eyes of many. One strategy is typified by immunization, which protects the individual, permitting him or her to survive in a dangerous environment and incidentally making the environment safer by reducing or eliminating carriers and vectors of disease. We see this ultimate outcome now with the elimination of smallpox. The other strategy, typified by chlorination, insecticides, and the Clean Air Act of 1970, aims to reduce or eliminate human exposure to disease by changing the environment directly, without adaptation or protection on the part of the individual.

The self-help and environmental approaches have many precursors; what is new is the widespread and even extreme nature of the vogue. Health food regimes and exercise programs predate recorded history. But now we have, or are establishing, credible statistical evidence of the consequences of individual behavior and environmental hazards. Changing lifestyles and environmental modification are both changing the incidence of many diseases. But it is the change in attitude toward the medical treatment mode that is most important for the future of health care personnel and institutions. The environmental strategy is a "social" approach, psychologically an extension of the technological fix through treatment; the individual is not expected to do anything, things are done for him or her, the environment is manipulated so that the individual is free to do as he or she pleases with less risk. Extremists among those favoring the individualist strategy would exclude some technology, such as drugs and immunization, but not other technology, such as vitamins and minerals. In one case the decision is placed in social institutions; in the other, in the hands of individuals.

Many plead for prevention under the misapprehension that it is a way of reducing medical costs. It is often said that an ounce of prevention is worth a pound of cure. The old prevention—clean water, sewage disposal, pest control, vaccination—greatly reduced illness and the need for medical treatment, at relatively low cost. It reduced total health care costs. But the new prevention, with the exception of clean air, has done little to reduce the overall burden of disease and medical needs, and at very high cost. In particular industries, such as coal mining, new requirements to minimize illness and accidents have made a big difference, but in the overall picture the new prevention adds hundreds of billions of dollars to health care costs (there are no reliable estimates for the total) with modest and declining contribution toward reducing morbidity and mortality. The age of public prevention has largely run its course, in terms of untapped potential for saving health and lives; microorganisms play a decreasing role in the agenda of medicine. We should be entering the state of behavioral prevention, at least until new research findings point the way for further contributions from environmental prevention and treatment.

Why Physicians Do Not Practice Preventive Medicine

Ah but they do! An annual physical is the typical example of what most people think preventive medicine is all about, but it is an early-warning device and no more. It never prevented anything; it only kept things from getting worse by spotting problems early. This is a considerable achievement, but it is not prevention. It is not even a good use of medical resources for people without complaints until close to retirement age. Likewise, the well-baby office visit is a device for early detection and may be useful in preventing more serious health problems and relieving maternal anxiety, but it is early detection, not prevention.

The closest most physicians ever get to prevention—apart from the frequent admonition to lose weight or give up smoking—is vaccination, which is prevention, typically required by law and usually administered by public health personnel rather than private physicians.

What people can do for themselves—diet, exercise, exposure to health hazards, response to stress, behavior toward risk—contributes more to health and longevity than all treatment of disease available in the medical armamentarium. Why, then, do M.D.s spend nearly all their time diagnosing and treating disease, almost none in improving the behavior and lifestyle of customers? This "lifestyle" aspect of prevention surrounds us: diet fads, exercise fads, miracle vitamin or mineral of the month "discoveries," sometimes with but often without a solid basis in research and understanding. This is not an area from which the M.D. is excluded from practice. Why doesn't he or she practice?

First, the training of physicians is oriented toward disease and treatment. This is also the expectation of customers. Few physicians know much about nutrition and its role in health and illness. A different medical education would be needed to concert the practice of medicine into concern with lifestyles as well as diseases and therapeutics. The dominance of specialization and the prevalence of referral to specialists might have to be reduced. Only the primary-care physician might conceivably look at a man or a woman whole; the specialists focus on a single function, a single organ, a restricted repertoire of technology. It needs to be added that what physicians or other health care personnel should learn and what they should teach is not settled (but then it almost never is, even in the conventional disease-oriented curriculum). There is much controversy on the amount and type of exercise to be recommended, on the value of tests on the basis of which doctors recommend or permit vigorous exercise. Nutrition controversies are legion. Better tools and more research are always needed.

Second, preventive medicine does not pay. Diagnosing an ailment, prescribing treatment, may be done expeditiously. The practice of preventive medicine takes a great deal more time. An M.D. cannot earn more than a fraction of the income practicing preventive medicine that he or she can earn in a normal practice; the preventive practitioner can see fewer patients, and will certainly have fewer patients, because few patients visit M.D.s when they feel healthy, and these few may be reluctant to pay more for an office consultation in a state of health than when troubled by pain or discomfort or anxiety. The physician must be acquainted with the lifestyle of the patient in considerable detail: physical activity, diet, work environment, leisure-time uses, the stresses to which the patient is subject and how he or she copes with them. Then the physician must recommend changes and persuade the patient to listen and follow through with them. This takes much time. A doctor's time is valuable, costly. The physician has not been trained for the preventive function; he or she is a disease fighter. The physician may be unfamiliar with the effects of the daily life cycle on illness and on health, effects that vary widely between individuals; he or she may not be adept at extracting needed information from the customer or at persuading customers who feel perfectly healthy to change their behavior in significant ways. The physician is not a salesman.

The suggestion that M.D.s become experts on nutrition, lifestyle, and other aspects of health maintenance is impractical. It runs counter to the seemingly inexorable trends toward narrower specialization. Nor is it apparent that a medical education is needed or appropriate. Specialization is driven partly by income considerations, partly by the M.D.'s concern for leisure and some control over his or her own life, by the need to keep up with developments in medicine. The explosion of knowledge in biology, the rapid evolution of medical know-how, the proliferation of tests and instrumentation, all rule out the prospect that many M.D.s can broaden the scope of their knowledge and practice while maintaining command in depth. The requirements for counseling individuals in seeming good health call for skills in interviewing and persuasion. Let us not fault only the physician for economizing time to maximize income, nor for the treatment mindset and ignorance of prevention. Most individuals without symptoms are never seen by a physician, limiting the scope of truly "preventive" medicine. The physician also realizes that there is a much better chance that customers will take the pharmaceuticals prescribed (although only half will do so faithfully), usually for a short period closely linked in time with the presence of unpleasant symptoms, than that they will follow a regimen of diet and exercise for years if not for life, during much of which time they will be free of frightening or unpleasant symptoms.

The customer, much more than the physician, believes in the germ theory of disease. The customer reasons in terms of linear causation, which is the typical way of thinking in American culture. He or she wants a positive diagnosis, identification of a specific cause, prescription of a pill or procedure. The customer is disappointed if the physician finds symptoms ambiguous, acknowledges that most disease will disappear shortly enough without treatment, that it is not always clear that medication should get the credit for self-limiting, self-terminating conditions, for the body's own ability to heal itself and repel invaders. Above all, many patients do not like to be told that their illness is really their fault, that the physician cannot dismiss it with a shot or a prescription, that they must be their own physicians and heal themselves. They often resent being told that they must revise their preferred lifestyles.

The customer, too, has to be reeducated before preventive medicine becomes possible on a significant scale. The individual motivation to follow advice is much greater when related to treatment of an existing condition than to prevention of a possible future illness. Smoking is a case in point. Everyone now knows that smoking is harmful; it does not take a physician to tell us this. Yet many millions (including numerous physicians) continue to smoke, and only the development of emphysema or a diagnosis of lung cancer will persuade some of them (even then, not all) to stop. Obesity is another example, recognized by all as harmful to health and attributable to overeating in the great majority of cases. Yet many not only continue to overeat but indulge in the theory that it is a disease, not a behavioral act, that there is a genetic predisposition to obesity. These responses relieve some individuals of guilt and responsibility, but not of hazards to their health.

Much of the advice that a preventive medicine specialist might give can be offered by information media. The role of the health professional is to provide encouragement and motivation, rather than information; for if the individual is adequately motivated and disciplined, most of the information is readily available. The role of Weight Watchers or Alcoholics Anonymous, for instance, is not provision of technical information and advice, but encouragement, support, peer pressure. The sources of information and advice to which we turn in health are very different from those we seek in illness. The sources are still physicians in many cases, but not in their private practice, rather via publications, radio and television programs, newsletters from various medical centers, and other information and education media. It is an educational task, an effort in persuasion, not treatment, nor even diagnosis in most cases. The plethora of diet books, for better or worse, is the health ministry of the future.

There have been significant changes in national diet in recent years, in response to fears of cholesterol and animal fat. Reduced consumption of eggs can be attributed largely to such concerns, whereas reduced consumption of some meats and increased consumption of chicken and fish (when it was cheap) undoubtedly was a response to price differences as well as health warnings. The vast majority of those who deliberately changed their diets were never urged to do so by any physician. The same can be said about the epidemic of jogging and other forms of tedious exercise. They were persuaded by the media.

The Demand for Environmental Modification

Why such a crusade to clean up the environment since the 1960s? The belief that smoking factory chimneys were harmful to health was well entrenched in the days of Thomas Carlyle, who was a crusader for clean air long before any of us were born. Consider also the drive for compulsory air-bag installation in automobiles (required by 1998), which are already equipped with safety belts. These currents of public opinion explain the negative reactions to President Carter's pleas that the nation meet the energy crisis by lowering its thermostats and follow his example by donning cardigan sweaters indoors. Change the environment, not behavior.

These attitudes may hail from earlier generations of colonists, settlers, pioneers, who fought a hard environment and gave no quarter. There is an enduring national preference for altering the environment to our will instead of modifying our behavior to suit the limitations of our surroundings. We accept no limits. Thus we invest billions in creating a fail-safe environment for accident-prone people, when a much smaller investment (seat belts, which must be fastened, versus air bags, which are automatic) would yield comparable results. AIDS has resulted in a great deal of discussion and considerable panic, but has not had much effect on the behavior of groups other than those at very high risk, and even then not a lasting effect. People want a pill, a vaccine, the chemical equivalent of medieval indulgences, or confession and absolution of sins, anything but even modest changes in behavior that would yield better results than can be expected from any vaccine or drug now available or in prospect. At enormous expense we create ramps to buildings, ramps on street corner curbs, so that the wheel-chair-bound can maneuver without assistance; we have altered some buses to the same end, even though at a small fraction of the expense we could have provided more convenient transportation for every wheelchair-bound individual to any place at any time.[5] To this same cultural obsession with untrammeled individual freedom we owe the diet pill industry.

Neither demand for nor supply of environmental health is individual. Nor in large part is it true of workplace and consumer product safety. Most prevention is provided wholesale, not retail. If there were an effective individual demand, much legislation and regulation, many new organizations, would have been unnecessary. People do not know most of the things from which they should be protected. And they have no choice: cleaner air for one is cleaner air for all. Laws and regulations are employed to preclude individual choice when it could be available: smoke detectors, air bags at the consumer level; and at the producer level the elimination of lead paint and CFCs in refrigerating equipment. Employers are usually insured against workplace accidents and some illness; so are workers, insofar as medical care is concerned. Neither is insured against environmental hazards, although medical costs may be covered by health insurance.

The demand for environmental and workplace protection tends to be excessive because the individual does not pay for it directly, only indirectly, through higher taxes and higher prices for consumer goods and services. By the same token, such protection is not concerned with achieving a given effect at least cost, requiring stack scrubbers on all coal-burning power plants, even though use of low-sulfur coal might be cheaper (eastern coal interests are involved here). Reduce air pollution everywhere, reduce radon exposure everywhere, even though most of the benefit could be attained at a very small fraction of the cost by concentrating on high-pollution areas.

With no concern for cost, demand becomes excessive. It is analogous to demand for health care with full insurance coverage. But there is something else: demand from those who do not stand to benefit, who happen to live in pollution-free areas, work in safe places, who thereby seek to impose the costs of environmental and workplace safety on others. It is as though demand for medical care came mainly from the healthy, not the sick.

What is the origin of demand? Mary Douglas and Aaron Wildavsky distinguish between two power centers: hierarchical organizations or government bureaucracies, and markets or individualism, and a third peripheral influence, the border or sectarianism, which accounts for most of the environmental health movement.[6] Each group selects its risks; each is biased in its assessment of its risks. The market concentrates on profitability and the short run; the bureaucracy is concerned with its stability and external threats. The border concentrates on long-term, low-probability risks; to give them credibility and urgency, it imagines threatening evil on a cosmic scale, sometimes described as "the sky is falling" syndrome. Douglas and Wildavsky draw an analogy between environmental sectarianism and Puritan fears of witches and the McCarthyism of the 1950s. Sects need to distinguish between the good people and the bad, whose concerns need not be protected; to develop the idea of conspiracy by the latter. The membership is constituted predominantly of educated, critical, articulate people with no commitment to commerce or industry, some of whom have figuratively replaced both Science and God with Nature. Most sects do not tolerate disagreement; they settle disputes by expulsion. Sectarians are antitechnology, anti-institution; they constitute a permanent opposition with no intention of governing; they dislike government and do not develop the capacity for exercising power. "The border tends to present humans as victims to be compensated and weaklings to be protected."[7] The essence of sectarianism is that demands are never satisfied; if one set is met, then new demands are escalated. The raison d'être is permanent opposition, therefore permanent dissatisfaction.

Needless to say this a somewhat simplified and exaggerated view, not applicable to all environmental groups. But it helps us understand why the war can never be won, why public agencies themselves, whether yielding to environmental lobbies or protecting their own turf, sometimes make unreasonable demands. To paraphrase Enoch Powell on health care, the demand for environmental health is infinite. It also helps us understand why assessments of risks and benefits by presumably competent organizations and individuals are so wildly different. In our present state of ignorance there is a great deal of uncertainty. Market-oriented groups, to whom costs are everything, will position themselves at one extreme; sects, for whom costs are nothing and risks are everything, will be at the other extreme, with nothing in common except a pretense or delusion of intellectual integrity. The choice of outcomes somewhere between is extremely wide and is necessarily a choice of values and political expediency, for where is the objective assessment? Thus we find legislated goals that are very costly if not impossible to attain, but not the funding or staffing to attempt implementation.

Environmental and workplace safety policies are entirely demand driven. There is no pressure from the supply side. Employers do not press for stricter workplace safety rules. (With high insurance rates or high cost of litigation resulting from work-related injuries or illness, there is greater employer willingness to accept OSHA regulations, that is, a derived demand for occupational safety.) The only supplier beneficiaries are firms providing safety equipment, but they have little if any influence on outcomes. The same is true on the environmental side: firms supplying equipment to clean up the air and water, providing less toxic pesticides, and so on, are the only ones on the supply side with an interest in increasing environmental health and safety. Most producers see environmental regulations as an additional cost and compliance burden.

The cost of environmental and workplace protection ultimately is not paid by the employer (although employers firmly believe otherwise); the resulting higher costs of production and higher prices of course are paid by consumers, many of whom are workers. How do we know this? First, profits of corporations, contrary to popular belief, are not large enough to cover all the costs of workplace and environmental protection. Second, profit rates have not suffered as a result of the large increases in these costs in the 1970s and later. A case in point is the pharmaceutical drug industry, whose costs were greatly increased after 1962, but for most years since that time has remained one of the most profitable industries in the country. Consumers paid via higher prices for drugs and a decline in the number of new drugs developed. All these costs were simply and quickly passed on to the consumer. As to coal-burning public utilities, their rates are set by commissions to assure reasonable profits, adequate returns on investment.

Everything is demand driven, but there is limited individual demand. If workers had to pay out of pocket (as they do eventually, but indirectly) for the additional costs of workplace safety, many if not most would strongly object. If citizens were taxed explicitly for the additional cost of environmental improvement, instead of having it borne mainly by producers in the first instance, many if not most might opt for the glorious sunsets that go with smog instead of paying the taxes and higher prices that cover the cost of clean air. Some would say that guaranteeing that water used for hosing cars, irrigating lawns, washing clothes, and bathing should be fit to drink is overdoing it; that air bags, much costlier than seat belts and providing only modest additional protection, are not worth the additional cost; that increasing car fuel efficiency to reduce air pollution, particularly in cities with low pollution, may beyond some point so reduce car weight that air-quality gain is countered by increased frequency and severity of injuries in car accidents; that elimination of pesticides and herbicides may so increase the cost of food and other agricultural products and reduce income available for other purposes that it is not worth it. The public is all for stack scrubbers on coal-burning power plants to improve air quality. But stack scrubbers (or other approaches toward reducing emissions) raise utility rates. If, instead, the public were faced with a tax equivalent to the higher utility rates to pay for emission reduction, all hell would break loose. But for single-issue activists and lobbyists, one can never do enough. Those who have made a career of complaining will not give up their career just because their initial demands have been met. The heroic ethic that counts no costs unfortunately is not very good at counting benefits either.

The Supply of Environmental Health and Safety

Environmental modification and behavioral modification are alternatives only in some instances. The community can make many changes in the environment that are beyond the powers of the individual, avoiding the need for behavioral modification, where this is a practical or cost-effective alternative response, which often it is not. This is precisely what EPA and OSHA are designed to do. We are concerned here with these new agencies regulating health and safety. The old agencies remain, but are subject to new requirements imposed on water supplies, garbage disposal, building safety, food supplies.

Environmental Safety: EPA

The mission of EPA is to protect the environment. It is concerned with a very long list of chemicals in the air, the water, the food supply, the soil, household products, and in the disposal of various kinds of toxic waste. Some of its activities, such as preserving the spotted owl, have nothing to do with health. Some have multiple objectives and hence cannot be judged exclusively in terms of their contribution to health. This is true of clean-air legislation. It does contribute to health but it also reduces the acid rain produced by sulfur oxide emissions from burning bituminous coal that damages forests and fishing in areas with acidic soil, that has destroyed marble monuments and buildings in Europe and the fountains of Rome by the same process, and that has rendered many buildings there and here nearly black that were once light and bright.

Most of its regulatory activities refer to substances whose effect on mortality is unproven, whose effect on morbidity is unknown and presumably small. True, for almost any substance of concern to EPA, one can find an anguished "the sky is falling" protagonist, but incontrovertible scientific evidence is missing. Often the attitude appears to be that if we can find no damage in 1,000 mice, it is only because we did not test 10,000. Or if people exposed to a noxious substance showed no sign of illness, it is only because they were followed for only five years, not ten or twenty. Granting that no one can prove a negative, this approach concedes that the case is weak. In environmental protection, as in medical prevention and treatment, there is a tendency to consider possible benefits, no matter how remote or uncertain, and to ignore costs, no matter how immediate or calculable.

The best evidence we have is on air pollution, especially particulates and lead, and on some carcinogens. Cancer is usually fatal and readily identified, whereas other impacts are hard to differentiate from the common run of illness and disability. Disability rates are affected by a very large number of variables, and it is devilishly difficult to separate the effect of any one variable, especially when variables interact (as do smoking and air pollution). And we are no longer talking about millions saved from illness or early death, but thousands, hundreds, even in single digits.

If benefits are hard to measure, costs are even worse. Unlike medical care, whose costs are borne mainly by a single industry bristling with reliable statistics, the costs of complying with EPA and OSHA regulations are spread through every industry and every household. The household may think that the price of gasoline has risen and knows that cars are lighter, but that is the extent of its awareness. Every industry bears some costs; those more heavily impacted may come up with estimates that, if added, would be an incredible total. They have an interest in overstatement. The Office of Technology Assessment, the Congressional Budget Office, the Office of Management and Budget have estimates for some new regulations, in advance of their implementation. Unfortunately, hindsight is much better than foresight, nor can these agencies be assumed to be always objective and dispassionate in their evaluations.

There has been a dramatic improvement in air quality since 1970, the year in which the most important Clean Air Act was passed (Table 11.2). The improvement is all the more impressive when one considers the substantial increase in population and large increase in GNP over this period. Lead decreased by over 90 percent between 1986 and 1987 as a result of eliminating it from motor fuels.

Table 11.2

Pollutant Emissions (10 million metric tons per year)

	1970	1991
Particulate matter	19.0	7.4
Sulfur oxides	28.4	20.7
Nitrogen oxides	19.0	18.8
Volatile organic compounds	27.4	16.9
Carbon monoxide	123.6	62.1
Lead	199.1	5.0

Source: U.S. Department of Health and Human Services, *Health United States 1993* (Washington, D.C.: Government Printing Office, 1993), 167.

Numerous studies have examined the effect of reduced air pollution on health and mortality. Douglas Dockery and others examined mortality between 1979 and 1989 in six cities ranging widely in particulate air pollutants, adjusted for smoking (which was more important than air pollution in explaining differences in mortality). They found that mortality was 26 percent higher in the most polluted city, Steubenville, Ohio, than in the least polluted cities, Portage, Wisconsin, and Topeka, Kansas. Fine particulates, including sulfates, were most strongly associated with mortality.[8] Frederick Lipfert, using a large number of variables, including several air pollutants, for 112 standard metropolitan statistical areas (SMSAs), illustrates how difficult it is to isolate the effect of any one.[9] Paul Portney and John Mullahy examined the relation between urban air quality (ozone and particulates) and respiratory disease, and found that a 10 percent decline in ozone is associated with a 15.4 to 16.4 percent decline in sinusitis. They estimate the benefit at $1.35 billion a year, whereas the cost of air-pollution control is over $30 billion. But there are other pollutants: sulfur and nitrogen oxides, and at one time lead, whose levels have been reduced, and benefits other than reduction of sinusitis. Particulates are associated with more serious respiratory disease.[10] Bart Ostra found a substantial effect of air pollution on loss of workdays and days of restricted activity among male nonsmokers.[11] Most studies compare morbidity, mortality, workdays lost between different cities for a census year. What we want to know is what happens in each of these cities over time—between census years—as a result of declines in air pollution. If cross-section comparisons are difficult, time series appear intractable.

We know that industrial activity in recent decades has generated carcinogens, most of which remain to be discovered. We have tested only some 10 percent of industrial chemicals so far. Regulations on the use of carcinogenic chemicals such as pesticides and herbicides have no objectives other than health. The problems are measurement and agreement on risk. We have only the poorest data on pesticide residues, not very good data on lifetime consumption. And estimates of risk are based on experiments with rodents, which are the best we can do, but not very good. Some humans are rats, but most are not. Experiments with humans are not allowed, and besides would take much too long (we can study natural experiments, comparing people exposed and not exposed to particular suspect chemicals). Rodents are short-lived; we can find out much more quickly whether they will develop cancer if they are given a pollutant found in water or food or air or a household product. The problem, apart from the species difference, is that they may be given the equivalent of drinking twenty gallons of contaminated water a day. In ten years humans would have developed cancer, had they not drowned on the first day. Or the animal experiment is the equivalent of eating 200 apples a day or scrubbing an entire stadium with a cleaning fluid. (There are a few tests in which different levels of exposure are used to establish thresholds for carcinogenic effect.) This is a quick way to establish carcinogeneity but not to measure human risks. Natural experiments—comparing rates of cancer in populations with quite different exposures—would be useful if we had reasonable data, which we do not have as yet, for pesticides (but we do for some other harmful substances).

There are large regional variations in cancer rates. The District of Columbia has the highest: 230 per 100,000; Delaware, Maryland, and Louisiana have rates over 190. Utah has the lowest, 124, followed by Puerto Rico, 129, and Hawaii, 138.[12] There are also large regional variations in the rates of specific cancers. These variations, which cannot be attributed to age or ethnic composition, indicate that environmental factors play a very large role, some suggest as much as 80 percent. (Others disagree. John Higginson, the original source of the estimate that environment accounts for two-thirds of cancers, objects that he was referring to total environment, including diet, lifestyle, and culture in West Africa; Philip Handler states that only 2 percent can be attributed unquestionably to environment.[13]) Accordingly, EPA has been active in identifying carcinogens and reducing their prevalence.

Estimates vary wildly. One estimate of the cancer risk of pesticides on tomatoes is 859 additional cancers per million; another is 0.32 cancer.[14] According to a National Academy of Sciences report, pesticides in common foods may cause 20,000 cancers a year. Foods with the highest risk include tomatoes, beef, potatoes, oranges, lettuce, apples, peaches, pork, wheat, soybeans, beans, carrots, chicken, corn, and grapes. Fifty-three pesticides have been identified as potentially carcinogenic. The conclusions were based on worst-risk assessments of twenty-eight pesticides: seventy years of consumption, maximum treatment of crops, and maximum residue.[15] (This is the same report whose estimate of excess deaths from tomatoes is 2,600 times that of another report.)

Cancer accounts for one out of four deaths, hence the concentration of concern on carcinogens. Much of it seems displaced. Bruce Ames estimates that the average ingestion of natural carcinogens is perhaps 10,000 times the weight of pesticide residues (but not of the carcinogeneity). Plants produce their own pesticides, many of which are carcinogenic or mutagenic. The catalog of plants with carcinogenic natural products includes most of the foods in our diet, such as lettuce, celery, mushrooms, beets, spinach, radish, rhubarb, coffee, tea, cocoa, herbal teas, black pepper, cottonseed oil, meat from animals fed on it, milk from cows grazing on a variety of carcinogenic plants, potatoes, corn, fava beans. Aflatoxin, a mold found especially in corn and its products, could be more carcinogenic than all pesticide residues combined.[16] Fats, including hydrogenated vegetable fats, also contain carcinogens. The process of cooking, especially browning and burning, and the caramelizing of sugar, create potent carcinogens. On the other hand, plants also contain anticarcinogens, especially antioxidants such as vitamin E, beta carotene, and selenium.[17] Manipulations by plant breeders to increase the resistance of plants to insects and other pests may add more to the carcinogeneity of our diet than all the pesticide residues. But are we going to give up cornbread and cereal and syrup? For the information of nonsmokers, eggplant is the vegetable with the highest nicotine content, followed by green and pureed tomatoes and cauliflower.[18]

I recall hearing a story long ago, no doubt apocryphal, of the devout Hindu vegetarian who looked at a drop of water through a microscope and found it teeming with microscopic life. Was he going to be false to his faith or die of thirst? Are we going to stop eating?

What is neglected is our exposure to neurotoxins.[19] Unlike cancer, they are unlikely to kill, only to diminish mental capacity and performance. How can we ever measure the effects or their elimination except in the most severe cases? Lead is the principal neurotoxin, and the spectacular reduction from the air and its elimination from paint is reassuring. But there are many others about which we know little.

Radon is considered by EPA to be second only to smoking as a (modifiable) cause of cancer. A study funded by EPA and the Nuclear Regulatory Commission concluded that it caused from 5,000 to 20,000 deaths a year.[20] Yet there is no conclusive evidence that radon at levels normally experienced is a risk at all. Two recent studies, one Canadian and the other

British, found no effect; a third, in Sweden, found a slight effect at expo-sures well above the average.[21] How could there be such a difference of opinion? The study finding thousands of deaths was not based on rodents but on uranium miners, whose exposure is more than ten times that experi-enced by almost anyone else. Then their experience was extrapolated to much lower exposures by using, we are told, sophisticated statistical meth-ods. Unfortunately, there is no statistical procedure that can tell us the shape of the dose-response relation as we move from very high to normal dosage, nor whether there is a threshold and what it is. The most common procedure is a linear extrapolation, which implies that a single molecule of radon, or of any carcinogen, could cause cancer.[22] We know this is not true; there are minimal thresholds; the body has defenses. And it is plausible that there is not a single threshold—that it matters whether it is exposure to low levels over many decades or to the same total exposure in a concentrated time period. (The problem of extrapolation to estimate the dose-response [can-cer] relation is found in animal studies as well.) On this flimsy basis, reduc-tion of the radon content of water in small rural water systems may raise family water bills $242 a year to save an estimated eighty-four lives (possi-bly a small fraction of this number) at a cost of $3.2 million per life saved (possibly a much larger cost).[23] The special problem of identifying the risk from radon is that it causes lung cancer, but the number of lung cancers associated with smoking is much larger; assigning cancers by cause is not simple.

Asbestos is considered to be next to radon in the number of deaths it causes. It can cause cancer, as well as lung disease, without any doubt.[24] Regulations to limit its use in construction should greatly reduce its conse-quences. But it is also found in some rocks, and since it is not a gas, like radon, does not dissipate as readily.

Other environmental putative causes of cancer are in the news from time to time and objects of EPA attention. One of them is dioxin. The issue is not whether it causes cancer, but whether it does so at the concentrations to which most people are exposed. The scientific community has not been persuaded that it does.[25] Another is EMFs (electromagnetic fields).[26] The fact is that we do not know very much about what causes cancer. There is a genetic component in propensity for many cancers. How important it is relative to environmental carcinogens remains an open question. If one excludes cancers caused by smoking, the rate of cancers has gone down. Compared to the environmental approaches a century ago, which added so much to life expectancy, the new environmental approach seems to be facing very small and diminishing returns and rising costs.

Even if we could measure the risk with some confidence, there is the issue of acceptable risk, which EPA assumes to be one extra cancer per million in a lifetime. Extremists say that it is too high a risk; others maintain that it is unreasonably low. By that standard, we would all have to give up automobiles (170 deaths per million in 1993) and electricity as well, never mind the combustion of hydrocarbon fuels.

Some would weigh the risk against the benefit (horse and buggy, kerosene lamps, and Franklin stoves are not risk free); others consider weighing benefits as unethical. In any event, it may be more difficult to weigh the benefits than to assess the risks. How much does the use of a particular pesticide (versus other means of controlling pests) reduce production costs and prices to the consumer? How does one compare lower prices and lower cancer risks? Given the lack of incontrovertible data and the diversity of interests—lower costs for farmers, profits for manufacturers on the one hand, commitment to a risk-free society and hang the costs on the other, and the poor researcher doing his best to get objective estimates in the middle— it is not surprising that the outcome is more likely to be political, another battle between lobbies.

Do not blame poor EPA; it is caught in the middle too, although its behavior sometimes suggests that it has been captured by the ecofanatics. So have juries, such as that awarding a plaintiff millions of dollars because her coffee was too hot. It is not surprising that some regulations run into many millions of dollars per life saved, much more than are found in medical care. EPA estimates of the cost to companies, public works facilities, and taxpayers of its regulations were $115 billion for 1990.[27] A less self-serving and more comprehensive estimate (which includes the activities of other agencies but is mainly EPA) was $500 billion—almost the same as the health care industry at the time. Its risk assessment of chemicals often exaggerates risks by a factor of 100 or more; it sets maximum concentration levels of zero for some chemicals not proven to be carcinogenic; it sets limits of one part in a billion or less for a large number of chemicals in water.[28]

If all requirements were enforced, the total would be much higher. An extreme case is the Water Pollution Control Act of 1972. "Based on the environmentalist's perception that pollution is priceless, the U.S. Federal Water Pollution Control Act of 1972 declared as a national goal 'that the discharge of pollutants into the navigable waters be eliminated by 1985.'"[29] EPA's own estimate of the cost of compliance was $317 billion in early 1970s dollars, which considerably exceeded the entire health care bill then, and would slightly exceed it today if adjusted for inflation. Often absurd if not impossible goals, combined with very weak enforcement, appear to be an equilibrium adjustment to irreconcilable interests.

How does one account for the wide variation in estimates of harm from so many substances? When data are poor, there is room for substantial differences of opinion. Beyond this, there is advocacy research and adversary research. Which estimates to believe? Frankly, all are in doubt. But I would place much greater credence on estimates published in leading independent scientific journals than on those of any organization, whether a government organization with a vested interest in magnifying its program or professional organizations and other special-interest groups with an interest in protecting their turf or expanding their agenda. We have seen some of this in the advocacy of questionable drug therapy and surgical procedures, but when outcomes are assignable to specific individuals, the room for imagination is limited; differences are small compared to those we find in the environmental arena.

Some claim that the greatest long-term threat to health is global warming, although objective scientists are not convinced that it is taking place. Those with long memories will recall that a generation ago the great threat was a new ice age, which again objective scientists were not convinced was upon us. Both warming and cooling are great threats? To whom?

Workplace Safety: OSHA

All OSHA activities are directed toward protection from injury and disease. One does not think of building-code regulations reducing risks of fire, or requirements for smoke detectors, or safety belt regulations for construction workers, or protective goggle requirements in many jobs, as preventive medicine. And medicine they are not, but prevention they certainly are. Where does one draw the line? There is no distinction between avoidance of accidents rather than of disease in terms of needs for medical care. And OSHA is concerned with both: asbestos workers and coal miners are subject to occupational diseases as well as accidents.

The cost of workplace injury and illness was estimated at over $116 billion in 1992 by the National Safety Council. There are less than 2,000 federal and state inspectors of job safety and health. Fines are too low, given the improbability of inspection, to serve as a deterrent. Anyway, one-third of industrial fatalities are motor-vehicle-related or murders. Many of OSHA's regulations are unrealistic and unenforceable.[30] Robert Smith found thousands of standards but limited incentives to comply with them, and no agreement on balancing health and safety against costs. He argues that more health and safety should not be forced on workers than they would be willing to choose for themselves if they had to pay for it.[31] (In fact, most costs are shifted to others who do not benefit, via higher prices.)

Again, unrealistic regulations poorly enforced, some sort of political equilibrium. I have just learned that restaurant workers mixing vanilla with dough must wear gloves and masks because vanilla is a poison, but I have not heard of any ban on consumption of vanilla cookies or vanilla ice cream. That will be the day! According to George Will, OSHA requires "Poison" signs where sand is stored.[32] Sand contains silica, which some think might cause cancer. Should we ban sandboxes and close all our beaches, or at least place "Poison" signs on them, and see to it that children build no more castles in the sand? Vanilla and silica are so absurd that they strike me as the work of saboteurs, not fanatics.

Work-related deaths have been declining since 1943, from a peak of 17,500 to 14,300 in 1969, the year before the birth of OSHA, rising to 13,000 in 1975 and 13,200 in 1980, then dropping steadily to 10,100 in 1990 and 9,300 in 1993. Deaths from occupational injuries are a more accurate, although much less complete, indicator than work injuries. Since 1980, they have declined in every major industry (single-digit standard industrial classification [SIC] industry).[33]

If we go back in time, we find a marked decline of injury rates well before the existence of OSHA, mostly attributable to company and consumer decisions influenced by legal liability.[34] There appears to be little recent progress by OSHA in reducing occupational injuries, with the exception of mining (Table 11.3). Smith examined the effect of OSHA on targeted manufacturing industries in the first few years. These were industries where safety hazards seemed worst, on which OSHA concentrated its resources, primarily inspection. Smith found the effects to be virtually nil.[35] Since 1980, rates in mining have gone down sharply, but there has been little change in other high-rate industries (construction, agriculture, fishing and forestry, transportation, communications and utilities, and manufacturing) or in wholesale trade, but rates have risen in retail trade and services and finance, insurance and real estate and services. In terms of lost workdays, only mining showed a drop. Injuries with lost workdays bottomed out in 1982–83, then rose; so did nonfatal injuries without lost workdays. The total number of workdays lost peaked around 1979, then declined slowly.[36]

Perhaps the situation is better than the numbers seem to show. There is fuller reporting; sick leave is more easily available; workers grow more hypochondriac. On the other hand, there has been a shift in the structure of the workforce away from higher-risk industries (mining, construction, agriculture, forestry and fisheries, transportation, communication, utilities, and manufacturing) toward lower-risk industries (finance, insurance and real estate, trade and services), which should have reduced all the numbers and rates (Table 11.4).

Table 11.3

Occupational Injuries

	1980	1990
Injuries with lost workdays (1,000)	2,491	2,764
Workdays lost per 100 full-time employees	63.7	79.8
Injuries per 100 full-time employees	3.9	3.7

Source: U.S. Department of Health and Human Services, *Health United States 1993* (Washington, D.C.: Government Printing Office, 1993), 168.

Occupational diseases are rarely within the control of employees; here the results look much better, and a better case can be made for policy guidelines. The plight of miners has improved greatly, and one can anticipate a great reduction in occupational diseases among construction workers (asbestos), painters (lead), and agricultural workers (harmful pesticides and herbicides). When we look at deaths from specific occupational diseases, there was a large improvement in silicosis: from 351 in 1970 to 150 in 1991. Coal workers' pneumoconiosis also declined, from 1,115 to 692 over the same period. On the other hand, deaths from asbestosis increased from 25 to 247. (These numbers are much smaller than the American Cancer Society's estimate of 9,000 deaths a year from asbestos, but most of the deaths caused by asbestos may have been reported as cancer rather than asbestosis.) Deaths from malignant neoplasms of the peritoneum and pleura remained unchanged, from 602 to 607, a decline from 8.9 (1980) to 5.6 deaths (1989) per 100,000 workers.[37] All of these occupational diseases involve long lags, so it is too early to pass judgment on measures to reduce their incidence.

Consumer Products Safety Commission

We turn now to injuries associated with consumer products. The progress is not impressive. The rate seemed to have peaked in the 1970s and fallen somewhat since. The rates for females are consistently lower than for males. Women are believed to be more careful than men. And they are less likely to use the consumer products associated with the highest risks of injury, such as workshop power tools and construction equipment. The main types of injuries, in descending order of numbers, are stairs, ramps, landings, floors; bicycles and accessories; cutlery, knives, not powered;

Table 11.4

Disability Days per Person

	Restricted Activity	Bed Disability
1970	14.6	6.1
1980	19.1	7.0
1990	14.9	6.2
1992	16.3	6.3

Source: U.S. Bureau of the Census, *Statistical Abstract of the United States* (Washington, D.C.: Government Printing Office, 1994), 136.

chairs, sofas, beds; nonglass doors and panels; and tables. These are all associated primarily if not exclusively with behavior, rather than with products. It is difficult to believe that injury decline has much to do with consumer product regulation. It may be attributable to the decline in the most accident-prone age groups, the young. As to types of injuries: falls, fires and burns, suffocation, and firearms are all down; the only cause that is up is solid or liquid poison. Total deaths, as distinguished from injuries, dropped from 27,000 in 1970 to 21,500 in 1990, then rose to 22,500 in 1993.[38]

What the findings on occupational injuries (as distinguished from illness) and household injuries associated with consumer products suggest is that they have much more to do with the behavior of the injured individual than with the characteristics of the products, tools, equipment with which they work. The theory of victimization, that manufacturers and employers are to blame, does not appear to be supported. The benefits of OSHA and the Consumer Products Safety Commission are modest at best. There is much to be gained by reducing injury rates. The lifetime cost of injuries has been estimated to be $158 billion for the 57 million people injured in 1985, $182 billion for those injured in 1988.[39] But more emphasis should be placed on behavior modification, less reliance on modifying products and processes.

One area that has shown substantial improvement, deaths from motor-vehicle crashes, may have resulted in part from changes in driver behavior, in part from modifications of motor-vehicle design, but the main cause is probably seat belts. These have been available for a long time, but were not used by most drivers and front-seat passengers until their use by drivers and riders became compulsory. The death rate from motor-vehicle crashes per 100,000 population declined from 26.9 in 1970 and 23.5 in 1980 to 18.8 in 1990 and 16.3 in 1993. This is important because in 1985 nearly half of accidental deaths were highway related (45,600 out of 92,500); only 11,600 were work related; and 20,500 were in households. Another 19,000 were public accidents.[40]

Some mention should be made of the FDA. It is one of the older prevention agencies. It is responsible for inspecting foods as well as drugs to assure their safety for human consumption. New technologies create new contaminants but also provide the opportunity for improved examination. Occasional scares, such as the recent illnesses and deaths from virulent *E. coli* bacteria in ground meat, will lead to more rigorous inspection.[41] What does it contribute? We would have to know what would have happened in its absence, and we do not know. It protects us more from the insidious slow poisoning that is harder to measure than the rare acute illness and death from poisoned shellfish.

Other organizations, such as the Nuclear Regulatory Commission and the Department of Energy, have a limited agenda in preventing accidents and illness.

Behavioral Modification

A megalomaniac attitude toward the environment has deep historical roots. Nevertheless, conservation also has a distinguished tradition, even if a less ancient one. Conservation implies behavior modification by the individual and by society. Trees are not all for cutting, game for shooting, air and water for waste disposal. The frontier is closed, and we are learning to live with limits. It is still easier to obtain public funds, or private cooperation, for an environmental modification approach (a vaccine, an air-pollutant standard) than for behavioral modification (avoidance of exposure, lower driving speeds). It seems fairer to impose the same changes on everyone, say, via fluoridation of the water supply, than to leave it to individual choice, offering an advantage to those with the knowledge, income, or both to afford equivalent protection via appropriate treatment. In particular it seems fairer when individual behavior affects the welfare of others, for instance, by spreading infectious diseases. Preventive measures by public health authorities amount to changes in the environment eliminating all sources of infection versus changes in lifestyle reducing the probability of spread.

It is now widely understood that health is largely within the control of each of us. The role of the M.D. in the administration of health was never as large as commonly assumed. The increased life expectancies in recent decades are partly attributable to increased care resulting from expanded insurance coverage and to the progress of medical treatment. But the reduced rate of heart attacks and strokes resulted most likely from behavioral changes: better diets, more regular exercise, and reduced blood pressure and cholesterol levels.

Prevention via behavioral modification is not supposed to work very well because the benefits are in the remote future, hence discounted, and the benefits are uncertain, discounted again. Costs (sacrifices of time, energy, sensory deprivation) are in the present and immediate future, all too painful. Individual prevention requires a very large number of deliberate actions or aversions—exercise, diet, sleep patterns, behavioral restrictions—carried out over many years if not a lifetime. The very small probability of significant gain or loss attached to single acts or aversions is psychologically equivalent to zero. The individual under these conditions is not risk averse, but risk prone. Why, then, should someone change diet to give up good things or give up smoking or not take it up at all in the face of peer pressure to do so? Why reduce drinking or adopt a regime of regular exercise? Thousands of doctors still smoke. There are reports that despite panic about AIDS, there has been little increase in the use of condoms or other changes in sexual behavior among low-risk groups, just a lot of preaching about it.

Some among us are risk averse, hypochondriacs; some are masochists, but not enough to explain the significant lifestyle changes in recent years. Could we be wrong about attitudes toward uncertain future benefits? I think not; we do not see a rise in the rate of individual savings and investment; on the contrary, savings have fallen in recent decades. What does happen is that individuals who would not repeat indefinitely behavior that is unpleasant eventually may learn to establish habits of behavior that are devoid of affect, which persist without need for endless motivation and determination.

My theory is that preventive behavior complements personal vanity in the form of a desire to be slim and trim, to exhibit good musculature, to perform well in sports. These benefits from good behavior can accrue fairly promptly, and with near certainty. So-called vanity cultures are expressed in speech, manner, dress. Our "me" generations do not differentiate by sex. There is much expression via dress: look at the bizarre attire prevalent among preadults, but more stress on conformity beneath the clothes. Why should the egocentrism promoted in schools (called "self-esteem") focus on the body? Perhaps because it cannot be hidden under the equivalent of Mother Hubbards, because it can be more evident more readily than distinction of the mind or character.

Substantial improvements in health and some increase in life expectancy are attainable, in some instances at very low cost, through prevention of accidents and abstinence from alcohol, tobacco, and illegal drugs. They cannot be prescribed. Can they be proscribed? We have tried without success to make drinking a crime. Reduction in highway speed limits, originally a conservation measure, but a major lifesaver, has broken down. Heroin and cocaine are illegal but in widespread use. Should we try again by criminalizing smoking? Seat belts are compulsory equipment on cars, but until failure to use them was made punishable, their utilization rate was under 20 percent. Should the population be compelled to perform calisthenics every morning, as the Chinese do, as many Japanese workers do? The issue is one of freedom as well as enforcement: freedom from the smoke of others' cigarettes, from the compulsion to use seat belts, freedom to do either or neither. One cannot open up the question of freedom without impinging on psychology, ethics, philosophy. Freedom *to*, as distinguished from freedom *from*, implies both options and free will.[42]

Nevertheless, individual behavior has reduced the risks of illness and accidents. Alcohol consumption has fallen. Americans cut down on cigarettes much more and much sooner than other advanced nations. Smoking-related deaths accounted for about one-fifth of all deaths in 1990, according to the Columbia University Center on Addiction and Substance Abuse. Smokers are down from a peak of 42.6 percent in 1966 to 25.7 percent in 1991.[43] Paul Leigh and James Fries found in a sample of retirees that no cigarette smoking or excessive drinking or excess body mass, and increased exercise and seat-belt use, resulted in direct cost savings of $372 to $598, and total cost savings of $4,298 per person per year.[44] Smoking and the overuse of alcohol and other drugs are draining Medicare funds. Medicare will spend an additional $1 trillion in the next two decades for people hospitalized by diseases caused by smoking, alcoholism, and drug abuse, of which 80 percent will be for smoking.[45] So the reduction in smoking and drinking is a major accomplishment. (The surprising fact is that after thirty years of unrelenting propaganda against smoking, so many still smoke.)

The proportion of Americans with high blood pressure declined from 36.9 percent in 1960–62 and 39 percent in 1976–80 to 23.4 percent in 1988–91. The proportion with high cholesterol dropped from 31.8 percent to 26.3 percent to 19.7 percent during the same periods. There has also been a substantial improvement in diet: less fat, less saturated fat, red meat, eggs (Table 11.5). It is surprising, therefore, to find that obesity, however defined, has risen, especially among the young. One-third of the population is now considered overweight, whereas it was only 24.9 percent in 1971–74 and 25.4 percent in 1976–80.[46] Lean cuisine must be a fad among the few. Americans with their cars, elevators, escalators, telecommunications probably did less exercise than most of their industrial counterparts, but in the past decade or two every city has witnessed an explosion of spas, health and exercise clubs, aerobic classes, and jogging, where once only the YMCA and YWCA existed. Mail-order catalogs and retail stores are full of home exercise

Table 11.5

Changes in per Capita Food Consumption

	Red Meat (lb.)	Fish (lb.)	Poultry (lb.)	Eggs (N)	Fats (lb.)	Dairy Prods. (lb.)	Sugar (lb.)
1970	131.7	11.7	33.8	309	52.6	563.8	101.8
1980	126.4	12.4	40.6	271	57.2	543.2	83.6
1990	112.4	15.0	55.9	233	62.2	569.7	64.4
1992	114.1	14.7	60.1	234	65.6	564.6	64.5

Source: U.S. Department of Agriculture, *Food Consumption Prices and Expenditures* (Washington, D.C.: Government Printing Office, various years).

equipment. Much is bought, but how much it is used we do not know. It is true that occupations have become slightly more sedentary on the average. Many elementary and secondary schools, their students and their parents, are obsessed with sports to the neglect of education—students are too tired and have little time or energy left over.

Although consumption of fats has increased (total fat content, including other foods, declined), there was a major shift away from lard and toward salad and cooking oils. As to dairy products, the consumption of milk and butter declined somewhat, cheese more than doubled, and yogurt more than quintupled.

This is Stuart Chase's Economy of Abundance, the consumer society, where self-indulgence is applauded and self-denial derided. At any point in time, tens of millions of Americans are on diets. Nearly all will fail; weight loss is soon regained. And most dieters, successes as well as failures, diet for reasons of personal vanity, which is a more powerful motivation than prospects of better health in the distant future. Jogging fads, aerobic fads, like yo-yos and Frisbees, come and go. Many who persist are masochists or narcissists who only pretend that they persist for reasons of health, and all too often injure their health. After all, man's natural state is a state of rest. And the cardinal sin of gluttony probably conferred an evolutionary advantage in the millennia of scarcity that preceded the rise of civilizations, as the sociobiologists must have concluded. So did individual fuel efficiency, which requires fewer calories to survive and function.

The advice the layperson hears on behavior changes over time. Animal fats are out, vegetable fats are in; oops! palm and coconut oil are out! Hydrogenated vegetable fats are as bad as butter! It's the amount of fat that counts, not the kind! If you drink red wine daily, most of your dietary sins will be forgiven. Diet will lower your cholesterol; no, for most people it has minimal effect. Vitamin C, or vitamin E, will cure your cold, or stave off aging. Do vegetarians live longer than carnivores? Moderate exercise or vigorous exertion? How much is actually known about the effect of behavior on health, and how certain is that knowledge? It is not surprising that people with long memories become skeptical of the latest advice, solution, explanation. How long before it will be rejected, superseded, even contradicted? Similar stories of stumbling from one half-truth to another by way of occasional error describe much of the progress of medical science (and science in general). But the layperson does not see it that way; in the quest for certainty he or she swings from one excessive expectation to another with intervening swings of frustration and skepticism.

The latest phobia is the depletion of the ozone layer and resulting increases in skin cancer. (There are other potentially more costly effects, but we are here concerned with health alone.) A vast propaganda machinery has been activated to eliminate the guilty chemicals from our industrial repertoire. At various times the hazard of the day was the mercury content of swordfish, the aflatoxin in peanuts, electromagnetic fields of high-tension lines, radon, lead, asbestos (the last two recognized evils), radiation near nuclear plants. Somehow, the dangers from radiation emanating from the millions of computer screens has never managed to become a national threat—neither did television screens.

Costs and Benefits

Everyone favors prevention, many under the illusion that it saves money, specifically medical costs. Sometimes this is true, but mostly not.[47] We favor seat belts because they save lives. Do they save medical costs? Does anyone care? Some end up bruised who might have been hospitalized. But others get trips to the hospital instead of rides to the morgue. Air bags definitely add to medical costs.

Many are disturbed by medical treatments that cost $1 million to prolong a single life for a year or two. This is very cheap compared to the costs per life saved of many environmental and workplace regulations. Supposedly we are always prepared to pay more for an individual life than for a statistical life. But that million dollars is for an individual; the $10 or $100 million is not for any particular life—it is for a statistical life. Comparing the cost imposed by EPA, OSHA, and the Consumer Products Safety Commission on the economy with the cost of the medical care industry, I am afraid that we are spending much more to save a statistical life than an individual life. This is suggested by Richard Wilson and E.A. Crouch.[48]

The Office of Management and Budget is able successfully to oppose proposed new health and safety regulations only when the cost per life saved exceeds $100 million.[49] The value of life is infinite, so some say; but saving 1,000 lives by this standard adds up to $100 billion a year; saving 10,000 lives would cost $1 trillion a year, which exceeds the total cost of the health care industry.

Kip Viscusi reports the following estimated costs per life saved of various safety regulations:[50]

Airplane cabin fire protection	$ 200,000
Auto side door protection standards	1,300,000
OSHA asbestos regulations	89,300,000
EPA asbestos regulations	104,200,000
Proposed OSHA formaldehyde standard	72,000,000,000

Back in 1981, it was estimated that OSHA's coke-oven emission standard would cost $4.5 million to $158 million per life saved; its proposed acrylonitrile exposure standard, $2 million to $625 million; and a proposed plan to reduce carbon monoxide auto emissions further would cost $1 billion in increased costs of production and would prolong two lives in twenty years. The Consumer Products Safety Commission's proposed lawnmower safety standards would cost $240,000 to $1,920,000 per life saved.[51]

EPA's expenses are trivial compared with the expenses its regulations impose on business, governments, and to a lesser extent households. Its failure to concentrate on measures that would save lives and prevent injuries and illness at least cost has meant that its efforts have accomplished less than they could have and have generated more opposition than they would have with a different set of priorities. The same criticism can be made of OSHA and the Consumer Products Safety Commission. A more compassionate approach would see their apparently distorted set of priorities as an outcome of the battle between risk averters at any cost and cost avoiders at any risk.

What the limited improvement in workplace and household injuries suggests is that the focus should be shifted to behavior modification and away from product and process safety regulation. Seat belts save lives, but they must be used. Propaganda helped in their use, but a legal requirement was more important. Drinking and driving is a risk that cannot be dealt with by mechanical solutions; education and regulation is the best approach.

Traditional public health policies for prevention saved, and still save, lives by the million. There is no need to count the costs. Most of the new public health measures save lives by the thousands, the hundreds, or in single digits. The decline in scale of prevention also applies to illness and injury. For this reason, it is important to give priority to the most cost-effective policies. If we were to enforce to the limit all the policies already in place, never mind many others proposed, there would be nothing left for us to eat.

Traditional prevention—safe water, vaccination—greatly reduced, and still reduces, medical needs and medical costs. These measures were substitutes for medical care. This is much less true of the new policies and not true at all of some. Another difference is that traditional public health increased productivity by avoiding illness at modest or low cost. New public health policies reduce illness much less and at much higher cost. Most of them reduce productivity either directly, by increasing costs of production, as do compliance with air-quality standards, or indirectly, by diverting too much of our productive resources away from productivity-enhancing uses. The rapid increase in medical costs as a share of GNP during the lifetime of the new agencies, although not necessarily attributable to them, is not consistent with the view that they save on medical costs or raise productivity. But we should keep in mind that our economic measures of output and productivity are limited: health, safety, quality of life are not included. Nevertheless, new public health measures compare unfavorably in every respect with traditional public health. This is to be expected: society deals first with the greatest threats and those that can be contained at lowest costs. Where to cut off—where to end the tradeoff between economic gains and other gains as the terms of trade grow progressively more unfavorable—is a political, perhaps an ethical, issue.

Cleaner air, pure water, safer workplaces, safer consumer products all contribute to health and life expectancy. In this respect they are no different from medical care, other than having an impact earlier in the process; they seek to prevent rather than cure. Their justification stands on its own ground. We do not chlorinate water or install smoke detectors to save medical costs, but to save lives. It is still pertinent to consider whether or not we are spending too much on prevention or making the best tradeoff between prevention and treatment.

It is not just a ranking of targets, but a choice of procedures to meet those targets. Air pollution, lead, asbestos standards save many lives or much illness. Radon is on less secure scientific ground. But even granting the case of radon, the procedure of inspecting every building in the country and setting a possibly unattainable goal of reducing and keeping indoor concentrations no higher than outdoor is absurdly expensive, whereas limiting inspection to high-risk areas would be feasible. The 1988 Radon Abatement Act goal of reducing indoor radon to outdoor levels might cost $500 billion. The EPA proposal to reduce radon concentration below 4 picocuries per liter would cost $20–100 billion. Fixing the 100,000 hottest homes, concentrated in areas with a high soil content of radium, would cost less than $500 million.[52]

How should we reduce highway deaths and accidents? There are many alternatives, not mutually exclusive. We could reduce speed limits and enforce them; everyone would be adversely affected (time is a cost), but there would be some reduction in air pollution. We could modify cars to reduce damage from collisions or crashes, making them heavier; everyone would be adversely affected, and there would be a slight increase in air pollution. We have required seat belts and their use; there was a small cost to nearly everyone. We can require air bags; the cost is much greater than seat belts, however, and their additional contribution to lives and injuries reduced is modest. The cost per life saved is estimated at $1 million.[53] We could raise the driving age, concentrating the cost on a few with the highest risk of accidents. We could cancel driver licenses for years of all those causing crashes, driving under the influence, or both, thus concentrating costs on those whose behavior indicates they are high-risk drivers. We have to consider driver responses in calculating benefits: seat belts and air bags may make drivers less cautious; so may heavy cars well protected against collisions. As for raising the minimum age for driving, is it just age or the fact that inexperienced drivers, whether sixteen or eighteen, are accident prone? Thus estimating benefits is not a cut-and-dried proposition. Costs, in contrast, are highly diverse; how do we value time lost by lower speed limits? The inconvenience of postponing or denying the right to drive? Or the distribution of costs, among accident prone and accidentproof alike, versus their concentration on the former? In making policy decisions, I doubt that all these alternatives were carefully compared, and priorities selected on a benefit-cost basis. Each policy has its avid proponents, its lobby. Victory goes to the best-organized lobby.

What does saving a life actually mean? We all die eventually. To make comparisons, costs should be expressed in terms of an additional year of life, a measure that also reflects the age at which a life is saved. That is one reason why vaccinations are so cost effective; for each individual life preserved, the average number of years saved could be seventy. The benefit estimates place far too much stress on lives saved, or prolonged, because they are much more easily measured than illness and injury avoided. In most instances, most of the benefit is in the latter. Cancer is the main exception, because of its high mortality rate.

Notes

1. Rene Dubos. *Man, Medicine and Environment* (Harmondsworth, England: Penguin, 1968), 103–4.
2. M. Harvey Brenner, "Industrialization and Economic Growth: Estimates of Their Effects on the Health of Populations," in *Assessing the Contribution of the Social Sciences to Health* (AAAS Selected Symposium), ed. M. Harvey Brenner, Anne Mooney, and Thomas Nagy, 65–115 (Boulder, Colo.: Westview Press, 1978). See also S.A.

Rudin, "National Motives Predict Psychogenic Death Rates 25 Years Later," *Science* 160 (May 24, 1968): 901–3.

3. Gregory Pappas, Susan Queen, Wilbur Hadden, and Gail Fisher, "Increasing Disparity in Mortality between Socioeconomic Groups in the United States," *New England Journal of Medicine* 329 (July 8, 1993): 103–9.

4. U.S. Bureau of the Census, *Statistical Abstract of the United States 1994* (Washington, D.C.: Government Printing Office, 1994), table 201.

5. Henry Fairlie, "We're Overdoing Help for the Handicapped," *Washington Post,* June 1, 1980, D-1.

6. Mary Douglas and Aaron Wildavsky, *Risk and Culture* (Berkeley: University of California Press, 1982).

7. Ibid., 190.

8. Douglas Dockery, Arden Pope, Xiping Xu, et al., "An Association between Air Pollution and Mortality," *New England Journal of Medicine* 329 (December 9, 1993): 1753–59.

9. Frederick Lipfert, "Air Pollution and Mortality: Specification Searches Using SMSA-based Data," *Journal of Environmental Economics and Management* 11 (September 1984): 207–43.

10. Paul Portney and John Mullahy, "Urban Air Quality and Chronic Respiratory Disease," *Regional Science and Urban Economics* 20 (November 1990): 407–18.

11. Bart D. Ostra, "The Effects of Air Pollution on Work Loss and Morbidity," *Journal of Environmental Economics and Management* 10 (December 1983): 371–82.

12. American Cancer Society, "Cancer Facts and Figures 1994," in *Washington Post/Health,* June 14, 1994.

13. Douglas and Wildavsky, *Risk and Culture,* 55.

14. Carole Sugarman, "Assessing Risk: A Risky Business," *Washington Post,* November 26, 1989, C3.

15. Michael Weisskopf, "Pesticides in 15 Common Foods May Cause 20,000 Cancers a Year," *Washington Post,* May 21, 1987, A33.

16. F. Aguilar, C.C. Harris, T. Sun, et al., "Geographic Variation of p53 Mutational Profile in Nonmalignant Human Liver," *Science* 264 (May 22, 1994): 1317–19; Leonard Stoloff, "Carcinogenicity of Aflatoxins," *Science* 237 (September 18, 1987): 1283–84.

17. Bruce Ames, "Dietary Carcinogens and Anticarcinogens," *Science* 221 (September 23, 1983): 1256–63; Lois Swirsky Gold, Thomas Slone, Bonnie Stern, et al., "Rodent Carcinogens: Setting Priorities," *Science* 258 (October 9, 1992): 261–65.

18. Edward Domino, Eric Hornbach, and Tsenge Demana, "The Nicotine Content of Common Vegetables," *New England Journal of Medicine* 329 (August 5, 1993): 437.

19. Sarah Williams, "Neglected Neurotoxicants," *Science* 248 (May 25, 1990): 958.

20. Marjorie Sun, "Radon's Health Risks," *Science* 239 (January 15, 1988): 250.

21. Richard Stone, "New Radon Study: No Smoking Gun," *Science* 263 (January 28, 1994): 465. See also Göran Pershagen, Gustav Åkerblom, Olav Axelson, et al., "Residential Radon Exposure and Lung Cancer in Sweden," *New England Journal of Medicine* 330 (January 20, 1994): 159–64.

22. Philip Abelson, "Risk Assessments of Low-Level Exposures," *Science* 266 (September 9, 1994): 1507. See also letters in response, November 15, 1994, 1141–44.

23. "Minimizing Radon in Water to Cost More Than Expected," *Washington Post,* April 3, 1994, A16.

24. B.T. Mossman, J. Bignon, M. Corn, et al., "Asbestos: Scientific Developments and Implications for Public Policy," *Science* 247 (January 19, 1990): 294.

25. Richard Stone, "Dioxin Report Faces Scientific Gauntlet," *Science* 265 (Septem-

ber 16, 1994): 1650; Eliot Marshall, "Immune System Theories on Trial," *Science* 234 (December 19, 1986): 1490–92.

26. Richard Stone, "Polarized Debate: EMF and Cancer," *Science* 258 (December 11, 1992): 1724. See also responses, April 2, 1993, 13–16. Gary Taubes, "EMF-Cancer Links: Yes, No and Maybe," *Science* 262 (October 29, 1993): 649.

27. Gary Rutledge and Christine Vogen, "Pollution Abatement and Control Expenditures, 1972–1992: Estimates for 1992 and Revised Estimates for 1972–91," *Survey of Current Business* 74, no. 5 (May 1994): 36–49.

28. Philip H. Abelson, "Pathological Growth of Regulations," *Science* 260 (June 25, 1993): 1859.

29. Yair Aharoni, *The No-Risk Society* (Chatham, N.J.: Chatham House, 1981), 60.

30. Peg Seminario and Peter Eide, "Is OSHA's Engine in Need of an Overhaul?" *Washington Times,* June 19, 1994, B3.

31. Robert Stewart Smith, *The Occupational Safety and Health Act* (Washington, D.C.: American Enterprise Institute, 1976), 2.

32. George Will, "Lunatic Laws," *Washington Post,* January 22, 1995, C7.

33. U.S. Department of Health and Human Services, *Health United States 1993* (Washington, D.C.: Government Printing Office, 1993), 137.

34. Lester Lave, "Health and Safety Risk Analyses: Information for Better Decisions," *Science* 236 (April 17, 1987): 291–295, esp. 294.

35. Robert Smith, *Occupational Health and Safety Act,* 67–71, 97–104.

36. *Health United States 1993,* 136.

37. Ibid., 137.

38. National Safety Council, *Accident Facts, 1994* (Itasca, Ill.: National Safety Council, 1994), 99, 102.

39. Wendy Max, Dorothy Rice, and Ellen MacKenzie, "The Lifetime Cost of Injury," *Inquiry* 27 (Summer 1992): 332–43.

40. Lester Lave, "Health and Safety Risk Analyses: Information for Better Decisions," *Science* 236 (April 17, 1987): 291–95; see also *Health United States 1993,* 128.

41. Robert Service, "*E. coli* Spawns Therapy Research," *Science* 265 (July 22, 1994): 475.

42. Henry Wallich, *The Cost of Freedom* (New York: Harper & Brothers, 1960), 21–30.

43. *Health United States 1993,* 156, 163.

44. J. Paul Leigh and James F. Fries, "Health Habits, Health Care Use and Costs in a Sample of Retirees," *Inquiry* 29, no. 1 (Spring 1992): 44–54.

45. Spencer Rich, "Smoking, Alcohol, Drugs Draining Medicare Fund," *Washington Post,* May 17, 1994, A7.

46. *Health United States 1993,* 166.

47. Louise Russell, "The Role of Prevention in Health Reform," *New England Journal of Medicine* 329 (July 29, 1993): 352–54.

48. Richard Wilson and E.A. Crouch, "Risk Assessment and Comparisons: An Introduction," *Science* 236 (April 17, 1987): 267–70.

49. W. Kip Viscusi, "The Value of Risks to Life and Health," *Journal of Economic Literature* 31 (December 1993): 1912–46, esp. 1943.

50. Ibid., 1912–13.

51. Gordon Crovitz, "Costs in a Regulated Society," *Wall Street Journal,* August 7, 1981, 18.

52. Anthony Nero, "Regulating the Great Indoors," *Technology Review* 97 (August/September 1994): 78–79.

53. Lave, "Health and Safety Risk Analyses," 293. See also Warren Brown, "Air Bag Aftermath," *Washington Post,* March 21, 1993, H1, H5.

12

The Demedicalization of Health Care

One of the topics in the previous chapter was behavioral modification: lifestyle changes in diet, smoking, drinking, exercise. In this chapter we look briefly at some of the things people can do for themselves in testing, diagnosis, treatment.

The positive feedback between an enlarged health care industry and a bloated definition of disease does have external limits. Like a pendulum, the more it swings in one direction, the farther it is likely to swing in the opposite direction. Many current varieties of health nuts, following the doctrine "Patient, be thy own physician, heal thyself," are harbingers of potential mass desertion from health care institutions and personnel. One can see an about-face in the medical profession, toward prepaid medical care, even to some halfway house to a nationalized system of health insurance, as a last-ditch defense of territory. Some of the increase in health care spending is only a transfer of health care from the household to the office and hospital. A reverse transfer is possible, desirable, and perhaps coming.

The Hierarchy of Health Care

The most common medication is self-medication. It is mostly used for minor ailments but is significant even for major medical problems. It cannot be proscribed or eliminated. It is the ultimate constraint on the monopolization of health care by M.D.s. It often means self-diagnosis and self-treatment, or self-treatment without diagnosis, in direct response to symptoms. It may also mean a follow-up on medical diagnosis and treatment under the instructions of a physician.

With illness, the first decision, whether or not to treat, is made in the household. If the decision is to treat, then the second decision, whether to treat oneself or to seek professional assistance, is also made in the house-hold. The importance of these decisions should not be overlooked.

One study found that three-quarters of illnesses and injuries are handled without consulting a doctor. In 60 percent of the cases, over-the-counter medicines were used exclusively, with usage initiated within four hours of symptom identification in three out of five cases. For cases in which an M.D. was consulted, there was a two-and-a-half-day lag from symptom identification to decision to contact a doctor and a further seven-hour delay before contact was made. Twenty percent of Americans use over-the-counter medicines (including vitamins) on a daily basis.[1]

The vast majority of ailments coming to the attention of the primary-care physician are not life-threatening; most of them are self-limiting, and most of them are self-terminating as well. For most ailments, the human body is the greatest healer; it needs little or no help, and much of what is given is to reduce discomfort and relieve anxiety. A very large number of complaints similar to those that occupy much of the primary physician's time are never brought to the attention of a physician. The proportion of such ailments left untreated, or self-treated by the sufferer, determines whether we are criti-cally short of primary-care physicians or have them to spare. This observa-tion is not limited to primary-care physicians. The caseload of many specialists likewise includes ailments that are not life-threatening but are self-limiting and, if not self-terminating, are largely incurable at present. Many of the chronic diseases and complaints of older customers fall in this category. Once an ailment or condition has been medically diagnosed, many customers can monitor their own condition, whether high blood pressure or heart problems or diabetes or asthma or any number of other ailments, without frequent visits to a physician.

Thus self-treatment, or more accurately, lay medication in the context of the sufferer's family, friends and neighbors, and the local pharmacist, has enormous potential for reducing the demand for medical services of many kinds, but especially those of primary-care physicians, and for reducing total expenditures on medical care. The extent of self-medication is a ques-tion of attitudes; information; medical supplies, drugs in particular; and cost, in time as well as money. Surveys conducted for the Nonprescription Drug Manufacturers Association in 1983 and 1992 indicate the dimensions of this hierarchy as related to drugs and show an increased resort both to nonmedical and medical assistance, as shown in Table 12.1.

The growth in third-party payments has radically altered relative costs of medical care in favor of recourse to hospitals, physicians, and prescription drugs, away from self-treatment, in that order, since the proportion of costs paid by insurers is highest for hospitals, less for office visits, least for

Table 12.1

Responses to Self-Treatable Health Problems

	1983	1992
Did not treat	37%	30%
Used a home remedy	14	16
Used over-the-counter medication	35	38
Used prescription medication in home	11	13
Called or visited doctor/dentist	9	17

Source: Nonprescription Drug Manufacturers Association, *Self-Medication in the '90s: Practices and Perceptions* (Washington, D.C.: Nonprescription Drug Manufacturers Association, 1992), 6.

prescription drugs (which, however, in large part are chosen not independently but as a by-product of office visits and hospital stays), and none at all for self-medication. The failure to make greater use of opportunities for self-medication as a result of the nearly free availability of medical services under Medicare, Medicaid, and other third-party payers is a major reason for the overuse of M.D.s, hospitals, and prescription drugs and for the resulting enormous and growing share of GNP going to health care.

Drug regulation in this country may be as unfavorable to self-medication as in any country, by restricting access to drugs without a doctor's prescription. (This is not to imply that there should be no restrictions on access to drugs.) The legal monopoly of the practice of medicine by licensed physicians, and the broad definition of what constitutes the practice of medicine (including the ordering of prescription medicines), reduces access to well-informed and even well-trained lay practitioners outside the health care industry.

Health care is not the monopoly of the health care industry or medical professionals. Countless laws and institutions are dedicated to preserving health, sparing the individual the necessity of becoming a customer of the health care industry. Treatment is always the last recourse of the sick (or the first of the hypochondriac or the malingerer). Prevention, which precludes the need for treatment, is the prerogative of the individual and the society in which he or she lives, not the health care industry. Information, provided by every medium of communication, by schools at every level, by many agencies both public and private, is required for effective prevention and successful treatment. Research, which seeks and often discovers new information improving the effectiveness of both prevention and treatment, is conducted by many firms and government laboratories, as well as by medical centers.

Demedicalization and American Values

The patient role is an uncomfortable one for an American because it conflicts with the prevailing system of values. The patient is both ignorant and dependent; he or she cannot be in control or exercise choice. But Americans value individual autonomy and see themselves, or wish to see themselves, as in command of their fate, as free to choose, not subject to irreducible uncertainty, to circumstances beyond their control, or to the decisions of others. It is not surprising that a good deal of hostility has developed, given patients' natural self-assertiveness. It would have happened even if doctors had not been secretive and often arrogant or condescending. Higher incomes, the cheapening of medical care through third-party payments, higher levels of education, and better access to independent sources of information have all accentuated the conflict between American values and the role of patient.

One expression of American cultural values is the demedicalization of health care: the shift toward self-treatment and alternative forms of treatment, for reasons other than the lack of income or access, and the greater stress on preventive measures carried out by the potential patient, who asserts control over treatment in one case, over health in the other. These tendencies are inevitable and need not be regretted except in terms of employment and income of medical personnel and facilities. It is not always true that he who treats himself has a fool for a patient. For one thing, the patient cannot so readily fool the doctor, if both are the same person. And preventive efforts are rarely foolish.

The average educational attainment of the adult population has risen from 9.6 years of school in 1950 to 12.7 years in 1990. It will rise further, as the less-educated older generations are replaced by the more-educated young. Now 85 percent of the population completes high school, and more than half of them receive some postsecondary education. One-third of the population of Washington, D.C., has a college degree. The college graduate has a different attitude toward physicians and health care than the individual who never finished high school or never went beyond it. The better-educated person sees the M.D. as a highly trained technician in a semiscientific field, no more and no less. Preoccupation with premedical and medical education results in the neglect of more general education and inhibits personal and social development in many cases. Doctors are no longer well educated relative to their constituencies in the way that teachers and preachers were relative to their constituencies in the past, when they too were held in awe. The decline in the relative prestige of M.D.s is only what happened earlier to schoolteachers, the inevitable result of the narrowing or closing of the educational gap between parents and teachers, patients and doctors.

But this is only one side of the story; an educated population is better informed and is trained to seek out information; and the growing market these people constitute has generated a vast increase in health information readily available at various levels of detail and sophistication. The variable most closely associated with health is not expenditures on medical care but expenditures on education.[2] It is certain that in the future the M.D. will be even less of a monopolist gatekeeper than he or she is now. This follows from the large and growing literature available to those who wish to treat themselves or their families, including sources whose sale to other than practitioners the medical profession once sought to prevent (and for a long time succeeded in doing so). A vast amount of self-help literature is being published, aimed at lay diagnosis and treatment, as well as at prevention and healthier lifestyles.

Resources for Self-Diagnosis and Treatment

What is to be done about self-treatment? Even television advertisements for nonprescription drugs intone that doctors recommend or use it, and add that "doctors know best." Should a systematic effort be made to inform the general population, so their self-treatment will be more judicious and perhaps reserved for conditions where possible harmful consequences of mistreatment are not serious and not likely? Or should every effort be made to prevent self-diagnosis and treatment? Prescription requirements for all pharmaceuticals would not prevent self-treatment with mustard plasters or ingestion of vast amounts of magical herb teas or apricot pits or seaweed or whatever is considered the panacea of the day. It would not prevent the harm that even "harmless" medication may do: preclude or postpone access of the customer to a physician who might be helpful. What many companies already do, that is, require a visit to a company medical officer or some physician approval as a condition of sick leave, avoids a certain amount of self-medication, but is unlikely that anyone, much less an American, would accept the degree of compulsion necessary to reduce self-medication significantly, and there is no evidence to suggest that this would be a good thing.

To provide more resources for self-medication, what is needed is a wider range of over-the-counter drugs and do-it-yourself test kits, and greater access to instruments that nonprofessionals might be able to use advantageously, given printed instructions. The average household has had a bath-room scale and a thermometer to diagnose fever as far back as most of us can remember. Cheap kits to measure blood pressure have been available for quite a few years, although most households do not have one. Kits to measure serum cholesterol have recently been made available.

Temperature, blood pressure, and cholesterol levels are the three indica-tors most widely used in physicians' offices. Will their availability in households diminish recourse to physicians? I think not, for people will become aware of departures from normal readings that would otherwise pass unnoticed. But they will have no need for frequent return visits for the purpose of routine testing.

Other equipment for particular illnesses is available, and more will come. Diabetics have had home kits to test for blood glucose for some time; they permit those who need insulin to time their dosage and improve the manage-ment of diabetes without frequent office visits for tests. Also available are peak-flow monitors for asthmatics, which reduce the need for emergency care; tests for pregnancy and ovulation; a test for the possibility of colon cancer (a stool sample is tested for blood). Also feasible are tests for nutritional deficien-cies (iron), syphilis, hepatitis, HIV infection, bacterial infections of the throat and urinary tract. In time, most of the blood tests currently done in labs will be feasible at home. Patients with renal failure do not have to spend long hours three times a week in hospitals for dialysis, nor do patients who need continu-ous intravenous medication have to be hospitalized. But these procedures are not as simple or as fail-safe as taking one's temperature.

This is the natural evolution of technology: first, at the hands of innova-tors, then of more numerous imitators, then standardization and routiniza-tion and growing accessibility. The druggist today is very different from the druggist of fifty years ago; today's druggist merely counts capsules and fills bottles with pills or liquids. His predecessor had a stock of ingredients and had to mix the proper ingredients in the prescribed proportions for each prescription. Formerly complex tests now come in kits; once innovative instruments can be bought in drugstores. Most surgery may be routinized, but must still be performed by trained and preferably experienced practi-tioners; but many steps in surgical procedures that once required skilled hands and minds can be done mechanically. Routine procedures have been monopolized by the medicinate.

Prescription and Nonprescription Drugs

A further step in the demedicalization of health care is a reduction in the list of medications available by prescription only. In most countries, many pharmaceuticals monopolized by M.D.s in the United States are available over the counter. This country has a better basis for demedicalization than most of the countries that make pharmaceuticals available over the counter. Nonprescription drugs are regulated by the FDA. Every drug is sold with a detailed description of dosage, uses, side effects, and counterindications, which is not true in many countries. The customer must be the one to detect side effects and counterindications. The M.D. may ask about them, usually on the infrequent occasions of office visits, but as we all know, the doctor asks only about a few, at best. Many customers rely on their pharmacist, always available, rather than seek information from their M.D., which is difficult to obtain by phone and not worth the delay and cost of an office visit. Since many side effects are rare or mild, it is best left to the observation of the regular user rather than the infrequent inquiry of the physician.

In 1972 the FDA initiated an outside review of over-the-counter drugs to confirm their safety and effectiveness, but also to consider the possibility of switching some prescription drugs to over-the-counter status. In 1991 the FDA established the Office of Over-the-Counter Drug Evaluation. In fact, more than 400 prescription drugs have already been de-prescribed. Peter Temin studied some of the effects, concluding that $1 billion was saved in the first three years during which hydrocortisone up to 1 percent concentration became available over the counter, and $770 million a year for the de-prescription of some cold and cough medications.[3] Potential candidates for switching include treatments for allergy, sinus, cold products, analgesics, antacids, and antifungals. Over-the-counter drugs account for about 1.9 percent of health care costs, about $47 per person per year.

There is always the danger of abuse of drugs with serious side effects; that is a main reason why many drugs are obtainable only on prescription. Of course, once obtained, they can still be abused and sometimes are. People use both aspirin and sleeping pills to commit suicide, and the fact that one is a prescription drug and the other is not does not really make much difference. Appropriate information on dosage and on conditions under which drugs should not be taken is already provided on the labels; the job is educating the user to read labels, making sure that descriptions are easily understood by someone without medical training or an extensive chemical vocabulary.[4]

Denmark and Italy have gone further in converting some drugs from prescription to over the counter. The big saving is in fewer routine visits to doctors.[5] What drugs are safe enough to de-prescribe? An established record of safe use as a prescription medicine is the best guideline.

A different problem is not the misuse of a drug by some individuals but the possible consequences for everyone, including those who do not use the drug at all. Antibiotics are the prime example of overuse, particularly in countries where they are obtainable over the counter, to the extent that their effectiveness has been rapidly reduced. Resistant strains of bacteria have developed. This would have happened in any event, but casual use, often for conditions not appropriate for the antibiotic used, accelerated the process. The use of antibiotics both for humans and for animals later to be eaten by humans (do they get prescriptions?) has also increased the proportion of the population that has developed an allergic reaction, particularly in the case of penicillin, eliminating it as a possible medication even when the bacteria remain vulnerable. M.D.s have contributed both to the development of resistant strains of microorganisms and to the sensitization of millions, but over-the-counter availability of antibiotics is the major factor in countries where they are on sale without prescription.

Computer Medicine

Nearly all homes will one day have a personal computer. Programs will be available to any household, both general-purpose diagnostic and for specific classes of health problems. They can be updated easily and as often as needed. Programs already available to take detailed medical histories will be mated to diagnosis and treatment programs. So-called expert systems will multiply, will be improved, and will become available. They need not be under the control of the medical care industry. One can visualize fierce competition, with one program developed by the Mayo Clinic available in shopping malls; others by Marcus Welby, M.D., or by "Bones," in drugstore chains or supermarkets; one by Dr. Spock in places where mothers of young children are likely to congregate. And of course such programmed computers could be available in rural areas remote from primary-care physicians. Although they do not make house calls, the programs are available day and night, Sundays and holidays included.

As an individual whose medical history is already in the computer memory (who may carry it on a floppy disc from his or her home computer) reports complaints, the program at various points will require inputs—instrument readings, chemical tests—whose results will be reported before it can make a diagnosis and recommendations for treatment or referral. It may be drugs, diet, behavioral change, or referral to a physician or specialist (or to a more complex diagnostic or treatment procedure). In addition to responding to information provided by the customer, computers could be designed to obtain some information on their own: they could be equipped with temperature and pressure-sensing devices and eventually with more elaborate diagnostic tools. Units located in shopping areas could also be vending machines, providing some medications, some tests. Technological and marketing ingenuity would find many ways to diminish the burdens on primary-care physicians.

One critical point in computerized diagnosis and treatment is the ordering of prescription drugs, or of tests and procedures that cannot be performed in the household or whose outcome cannot be interpreted by a layperson. At that point, the individual's desire for self-management comes into conflict with the M.D.'s professional interest in health care. In most such cases the program should advise contacting a physician or appropriate specialist. How may this process of self-medication drawing on the knowledge and experience, not of specific M.D.s, but some of the best in the profession, be facilitated? Some relaxation of the physician's stranglehold on access to prescription drugs, some reclassification of drugs as for sale under prescription only, could be accomplished.

The individual might obtain direct access to commercial laboratories and testing facilities, instead of depending on the doctor or the hospital as intermediaries. A person does not have to become knowledgeable; the computer program can interpret the test results. Lastly, greater use could be made of physician-extenders and substitutes, such as physician assistants, nurse practitioners, nurses, and other paramedical personnel, many of whom were trained at a time when there was a perception of physician shortage and some of whom are considered expendable now that shortage has become surplus. Their help is seen as less threatening to individual autonomy than institutional care. They can assist the individual who wishes to exercise control over care instead of extending the physician's services.

A second critical point is access to a physician when this is called for. The general practitioner or other primary-care physician performs two functions: diagnosis and either treatment or referral. The customer relies on the general practitioner or internist to determine whether or not a specialist is needed, and if so, what kind of specialist, and further recommends a specific individual. How can this referral function be circumvented? Strictly speaking, all physicians could be the first point of access to medical care, provided a diagnosis has pointed to their specialty. The computer program can do all this except recommend a specific individual; it can list appropriate specialists in any area. (One can imagine programs charging specialists for inclusion in the list.) The customer may of course go through the Yellow Pages or consult the local medical society and obtain names. But how does the customer obtain additional information on the basis of which he or she can make a more informed choice? Someday we will be able to subscribe to medical rating services, comparable to the bond rating services whose results are free for all.

Alternative Medicine?

So far, demedicalization has been described in terms of shifting responsibility and decision making from medical practitioners to customers, using some of the same information, the same tests, diagnostic techniques, and medication monopolized by physicians. There is another meaning to demedicalization: recourse to alternative practitioners and alternative therapies. An Office of Alternative Medicine was established in 1991 within NIH and apparently is still experiencing birth pangs.[6]

As mentioned in Chapter 7, various ethnic groups have a tradition of folk medicine that is still alive in this country. And there are therapies for specific conditions, some of which are being incorporated into standard medical practice, such as massage for physical rehabilitation, acupuncture for riskless anesthesia. Other practices are more comprehensive, such as homeopathy, which is quite common in Europe. This topic lies beyond our scope. But there is no indication that demedicalization in this country is likely to proceed via adoption of alternative therapies or greater resort to nonmedical practitioners (psychological problems aside).

Demedicalization of health care is the result of a growing belief in lifestyle as a determinant of health; a desire to keep one's health under one's own control; better information as a basis for choice and action; fear of treatment, surgery especially; some loss of faith in the medical industry; and a growing repertoire of test kits, diagnostic instruments, and over-the-counter drugs.

Notes

1. Bruce Yandle, *Regulated Advertising and the Process of Self-Medication* (Washington, D.C.: Proprietary Association, 1980).

2. Richard Auster, Irving Leveson, and Deborah Sarachek, "The Production of Health, an Exploratory Study,"*Journal of Human Resources* 4 (Fall 1969): 412–36.

3. Peter Temin, "Costs and Benefits in Switching Drugs from Rx to OTC," *Journal of Human Resources* 18 (Spring 1983): 187–205; Peter Temin, "Realized Benefits from Switching Drugs," paper, September 1990.

4. Various surveys suggest that the problem is exaggerated; consumers read labels carefully and their knowledge of over-the-counter medicines compares favorably with their knowledge of nutrition, banking, insurance, and much other information. Also, they rarely exceed the recommended dosage or time limits recommended. Reported in Nonprescription Drug Manufacturers Association, *Self Medication's Role in U.S. Health Care* (Washington, D.C.: Nonprescription Drug Manufacturers Association, 1993), 5.

5. "A Prescription for Change," *The Economist,* November 7, 1992, 20.

6. Eliot Marshall,"The Politics of Alternative Medicine" *Science* 265 (September 30, 1994): 2000–2002; Natalie Angier, "U.S. Head of Alternative Medicine Quits," *New York Times,* August 1, 1994, A12.

13
What to Do?

Previous chapters have outlined *why* radical changes have to be made, and will be made, in the health care system, preferably early and calmly, but more likely late and with much sound and fury and lasting social disruption. In this chapter I discuss *what* must be done. I do not attempt to propose *how* it should be done. If war is too important to be left to the generals, health policy is too important to be left to the medical care industry; that is how we got into our present fix. It took decades to arrive here; it cannot be corrected quickly.

What Health System Do We Want?

Reining in health care spending is not an end in itself, only a means toward other ends. So first, what are our goals, what kind of health system do we want? I propose the following goals:

1. Provide universal coverage for health care meeting minimum standards of need and treatment; we are the only advanced nation that does not do this. Curtailment of spending should not be at the expense of this goal.
2. Reduce the share of GNP spent on health care. There is no need to spend twice as large a share of GNP on health care as some advanced countries with universal coverage and better outcomes in terms of infant mortality and life expectancy at every age.
3. Reduce the future increase in share of GNP spent on health care. Some increase is essential to care for an aging population. The effect of technologies yet to be developed cannot be predicted but can be influenced. It is unthinkable that within the lifetime of most of us, we should be devoting one-third of GNP to medical care, which is the implication of current trends. This goal, together with the second goal, seeks to preserve growth opportunities for the economy and maintain and improve people's standards of living.

4. Provide more information and resources to improve individual efforts in prevention, self-treatment, and home care, thus reducing the need and demand for medical care. But let us not delude ourselves into thinking that more prevention and home care are an answer to the problem of high and rising costs.

5. Improve knowledge about the costs and consequences of public measures to promote a healthy environment. We need better information to compare the effectiveness and cost of prevention versus treatment and of public versus private preventive measures, if we are to make the best use of resources to promote health.

Most people will accept these goals. But it is not enough to list goals; one must also establish priorities and give relative weights, since not everything can be done at once; and we have not specified how far to go, especially with regard to goals 1 and 2. One might argue that it is more important to slow down the rate of increase in health care costs in the long run than to reduce the level of costs now. Stress on reducing the rate of growth in health expenditures can eventually achieve the same result as lowering the level of the base, but the impact on losers will be stretched out. For there are losers, who will strongly oppose efforts to contain costs in the present and their growth in the future. Yet, if we do not get the base level of costs down soon, the rate of increase will be higher because the pace of economic growth will be slowed by diversion of large resources from growth-inducing activities to health care. The minimum target of health care reform should be an annual percentage increase in total health care costs not greater than the percentage increase in GNP. This total includes both price increases and increases in quantity of services. Eventually, health care cost increases should be less than the increase in GNP, reducing health care as a percentage of GNP.

Policies can be divided into two parts: those designed to lower the base of health care costs, but that would not result in continuing reductions, and those designed to slow or reverse the rate of increase. Lowering many prices, many earnings, reducing administrative costs, and reducing the quantity of many tests and procedures are once-and-for-all approaches toward lowering the base. So is cutting back on medical school enrollments and the employment of immigrant M.D.s, although the initial impact would be to raise costs and the base-lowering effect would take decades to work itself out. Measures to reduce the rate of increase on a long-term if not permanent basis would include limiting the scope of insurance coverage and possibly the level of reimbursement; redirecting research toward cost-reducing technologies; and limiting approval and coverage of halfway technologies that add to costs and do little for health.

Any honest program to lower costs and slow their rate of increase will cost many jobs, certainly over a million, perhaps many more. Most of the insurance companies' 268,000 employees would go, as would a sizable proportion of the administrative employment in hospitals and other providers of health services. There would be losses among health care personnel as well, perhaps substantial losses. And it would lower many incomes.

We should take a close look at the health system we have and ask whether, for the resources we spend on it, it is the best we can get. One needs to concentrate, first, on the principal causes of mortality and morbidity. One should not ignore the kind of life that is prolonged. If prolonging life adds to the sum total of morbidity, it becomes another cost of medical care. It is necessary to consider, second, the extent to which these causes can be reduced by intelligent and organized activity; third, the most effective approach, to the extent that there are alternative therapeutic and/or institutional approaches; and finally, the organizational, educational, occupational implications of one's choices.

Infant mortality is considerably higher in the United States than in a number of other advanced nations. The single most important cause today appears to be the lack of prenatal care. Drinking, smoking, drug taking, and maternal malnutrition may all be contributory factors. For children and young adults, accidents are the major cause of death. Nearly half of all accidental deaths are automobile related. Drugs are a significant cause of death among teenagers and young adults. Violent deaths—murder, suicide, accidents—again often drug- or alcohol-related, are the main source of mortality during the young and middle adult years.

A health care system directed at reducing mortality and morbidity among older children and young adults should be targeted on drinking, drugs, driving, nutrition, and mental health (and smoking, although its effects are likely to be long delayed). This of course is a health care system vastly different from the one we have today. A system aimed at reducing mortality and dealing with morbidity among the old should focus primarily on cancer, heart disease, strokes, diabetes, Alzheimer's disease, osteoporosis. This comes closer to what our present health care system spends its time and resources doing, but it is not doing it very effectively. Progress on most cancers is glacier slow, nearly all gains are from earlier detection and treatment. More has been achieved for heart and stroke victims with new surgical techniques, and for those prone to heart attacks and strokes, with changes in nutrition and the use of preventive drugs. The best prospects lie in prevention in both cases, rather than in treatment, and prevention is an environmental issue to a considerable extent in the case of cancer, a behavioral matter in the case of stroke and heart disease. Alzheimer's regrettably is still a subject for research, not for treatment or prevention. So is AIDS.

How Much Should We Spend?

How much we should spend on medical care is a subject of enormous complexity. We do not pretend to provide an answer, only to suggest subsidiary questions and survey some of the unsolved, perhaps insoluble, issues involved. In the long run, with changes in technology and longevity, we cannot say what should be the appropriate share of GNP devoted to health; it should rise, but not from a current base that is greatly inflated, nor from excessive increases in prices and quantities of services.

First, what prices should we pay for medical care? The answer, for most prices, is, much lower than we pay now. Earnings of a large proportion of health care personnel have risen out of line with earnings in general, especially in the case of specialist M.D.s. Their earnings should be lowered until those of primary-care physicians become competitive with them. Reducing earnings to where they stood relatively in, say, 1960 would lower fees and hospital operating costs (60 percent of which are for labor) significantly. Other charges, especially in hospitals, should be reduced by avoiding duplication of expensive equipment and services and by reducing hospital excess capacity—all this without reducing the quantity of services provided.

How much reduction in quantity should there be in tests, procedures, surgery? Agreement on this question may be impossible. How much should be spent on very underweight newborns sentenced to a life of serious disability and dependency should they survive at all? Most of the ensuing lifelong costs are not included in health care costs but nevertheless are attributable to extraordinary health care measures taken in the first few months. If a family wishes to bear these costs, and is fully informed about them, it has the right. But it has no right to impose these costs on the rest of us as taxpayers and as payers of insurance premiums. A bigger issue is the cost of dying. Nearly one-third of all medical costs are incurred in the last year of life. Even those who instinctively cringe at the thought of cost-benefit analysis have to recognize that this is too much. How much should be spent on the terminally ill, on extending briefly the life of the very elderly whose condition offers no hope of functional recovery? On the costly ailments of AIDS patients with a life expectancy of months or at best a year or two, even if treated at great expense?

How much is a life worth? How much should be spent on medical care in order to save a life? Many find such questions objectionable. They do not wish to consider lives in monetary terms, but do not hesitate to spend other people's money. They do not want to admit that a life saved at age ten is worth more than one saved at age eighty, even though the former means ten times as many years of expected life saved. The "right" to almost unlimited amounts of health care is a very recent invention. How and why it came about I am not sure. It is part of the shift in cultural values from individual duties and responsibilities to individual "rights" and self-expression carried to such an extreme that it runs roughshod over more traditional rights of other individuals. But when insurance premiums have to cover the extension of "rights" to health care beyond the limits most policyholders would consider reasonable, and particularly when insurance coverage itself becomes compulsory, then it amounts to taxation without representation.

How much health care is enough? What health status is adequate? There is a social consensus that no one should go hungry; everyone should have an adequate supply of food, and a nutritionally adequate diet. But no one is entitled to caviar, champagne, or lobster. The programs we have for supplying food to the poor are limited, not open-ended. Those who wish caviar, and can afford to pay for it, will eat it; others will not. The same situation must prevail in medical care. There is a consensus that everyone should have essential medical care, but unlike nutritional requirements, some need no medical care, others need a great deal. And third-party payments cannot be rationed in the way food stamps are rationed. What is "need," and how much of it is there? There is great reluctance to accept the fact that there is not enough medical care to meet all needs, there never will be, and perhaps it does not matter very much anyway, so far as health status is concerned.

Doctors and hospitals, the traditional health care industry, are diminishing in importance in the management of health. By now the major, and still increasing, share of their role is dealing with the failures of prevention, information, and self-care. How much should we spend on medical care? What ratio of M.D.s to population should we have? Neither question makes any sense without reference to what is being done, to what can be done, by means other than treatment. The optimal amount to spend on medical care depends on how much need for medical care is preempted by effective prevention via environmental control and via behavior-lifestyle choices. How much is accomplished by these methods depends in turn on knowledge generated by research and information about this knowledge conveyed to the population as custodians of their own health and to representatives of the community as their agents for the common good acting through the legislative and executive branches of government. How much medical treatment can accomplish that was not or could not be accomplished through preventive means depends on the contribution of research to understanding the causes of disease and finding ways of eliminating the causes or counteracting their effects.

How much to spend depends ultimately on the productivity of medical care. It is low and perhaps declining; one reason we spend too much.

Currently it is lowered by a large surplus of M.D.s, hospital beds, equipment, which result in excess supply of tests, services, and procedures. We can raise productivity by cutting spending in the right way.

We outline below what must be done to attain several and somewhat conflicting goals. We do not propose to suggest how it is to be accomplished. Agreement on broad goals is easy; on the choice among policies and policy instruments, it is impossible. First on the agenda must be manpower.[1]

Medical Manpower

As long as providers can profit by rendering more services, they will tend to offer more than can be medically justified. If there is an excess supply of providers and facilities, their influence will be reflected in additional demand from customers. With health care insurance, too much will be demanded.

A first necessary step is reform in manpower policy. Medical school output, some 16,000 a year, must be cut drastically and for a long time to come. The surplus of physicians drives prices and the quantity of services up and up. It will take decades to undo the excesses of the previous generation. How much to cut depends on what penalty we are willing to impose on the next generation of would-be doctors to correct for the excesses of the past. Unfortunately there is no such thing as intergenerational equity. The more we cut, the quicker the adjustment. How to cut? Several dozen mediocre medical schools should be closed, but the obsession with "fairness" suggests cuts across the board instead. This will mean temporary increased labor costs for hospitals, which experience a reduction in cheap interns and residents (to be dealt with by other policies). Hospitals will predictably seek to import more foreign medical graduates to fill the gap. The problem is not just the inflow, but the fact that most who enter stay. Import of foreign physicians to provide relatively cheap labor for hospitals and managed-care organizations should be ended, without eliminating the possibility of immigration for experienced and highly regarded foreigners.

Since we have no control over the number of Americans trained in foreign medical schools, it will be necessary to restrict if not eliminate their entry into the practice of medicine in this country. This will be necessary because with any substantial cut in medical school enrollments in this country, the number of Americans going to foreign medical schools will rise sharply. This will have to be done with substantial advance warning, so as not to penalize those already in foreign medical schools. Temporary exceptions could be made for general practice and specialties in short supply. A decline in the surplus of specialists should make it less painful to cut prices and fees inasmuch as the amount of services rendered per specialist would increase. Of course, previous increases in surplus, which should have lowered prices if there had been such a thing as price competition, did exactly the opposite. So do not count on price moderation on physicians' own accord.

Another consideration in deciding how much to cut is the need to increase, not reduce, the number of general practitioners coming out of medical schools and entering residencies. An alternative policy is relaxing the restrictions on the practice of registered nurses and other highly trained specialists. This should be done in any case as a stopgap while the number of generalists is increased, and as a long-term policy to reduce the labor costs of medical care, since much work done not only by generalists but by some specialists could be handled by suitably trained technicians, nurses, and physician assistants. The monopoly position of M.D.s is almost unique in the world of labor and helps account for excessive fees and earnings.

Medical schools have every incentive to maintain their enrollments, and institutions no less than individuals cling to life as long as possible. Hospitals have every incentive to maintain and even increase their employment of interns and residents, including foreign medical graduates. It will not be easy or quick to overcome these counterproductive incentives.

Since avuncular advice from former HEW secretary Joseph Califano and others has failed to accomplish anything, the job will have to be done through the price system, through powerful incentives and deterrents. All subsidies to medical schools, students, interns, and residents should be terminated, temporarily raising costs of medical education and hospital care. The gap in income between primary-care physicians and specialists must be closed. None of this will help reduce regional disparities. One can argue that residents of remote areas have no more "right" to a full range of medical services than to an excellent college or fine French restaurant.

Most of the medical care available for the next generation will be delivered by physicians who have long since completed their medical education. The long working life of any occupation is a problem whenever the requirements for that occupation are undergoing considerable change. Under such circumstances, education cannot be limited to the new generation of M.D.s. It is a problem also in changing medical school and internship programs; such changes will lack the heartfelt support of much medical school faculty, themselves the products of a tradition that needs reconsideration. Beyond medical education, the matter of licensing needs major revision, both in scope and duration. The range of activities over which licensed M.D.s have exclusive jurisdiction needs to be narrowed, to recognize the proper role of nurse practitioners, registered nurses, physician assistants, as well as clinical psychologists, acupuncturists, and other specialists currently regarded as beyond the pale who have a contribution to make. Second, the practice of granting the same broad license to practice to all M.D.s makes no sense in view of their often narrow specialization. Board certification de facto may limit the license to practice a specialty in many cases, but this de facto approximation should become de jure. Why should a surgeon retain the right to general practice? Third, given the rapid evolution of knowledge and standards, no license should be granted for life. If a driver has to be reexamined periodically to retain his license, why not an M.D., to ascertain that he has kept up with his field and can practice today's medicine, not only what he learned in medical school and internship? If licenses were restricted by specialty, and limited to a finite number of years, then appropriate provision would have to be made, not just for relicensing, but for the retraining and updating to justify it.

While considering manpower, let us not neglect medical education. It is a long, wasteful, and expensive process, a vested interest of medical school and faculty and teaching hospitals. It has not adjusted to the fact that the vast majority of practicing physicians are specialists, many very narrow specialists, who can use only a small part of all they were taught in medical school and who promptly and properly forget most of the rest. It concentrates unduly on ailments rarely encountered by most practicing physicians and gives little attention to the patient as a human being.[2] In a 1979 article in the *Washington Post*, former *Science* news editor Daniel Greenberg concluded that "we have heavily goldplated the medical education system, so that, in terms of what most doctors do most of the time, their long and costly training is rarely relevant. . . . The present medical education system is akin to putting all bus drivers through astronaut training."[3]

There are numerous suggestions for the reform of medical schools, and some efforts in that direction, which should shorten medical education for most and reduce its costs, and thereby the debts of new graduates and the argument that high earnings of doctors who graduated long ago are justified by the high debts of those who graduated yesterday. Another example of intergenerational injustice.

Narrower specialization along the same lines as before may not be the answer for tomorrow. There are enough problems now with patients whose needs do not fit neatly within the blindered perspective or selective knowledge of particular specialists. A reconsideration of medical education in terms of scientific advances and changes in the place of physicians in health care and the organization of health care delivery is overdue. The kinds of people selected for medical school, the process of medical education, and the subsequent process of training and apprenticeship depend on the future functions of physicians. Currently most specialties are characterized by a drawing and quartering process: ear, nose, and throat; ophthalmology; cardiology; dermatology; gastroenterology; obstetrics and gynecology; urology. Some are by disease group (e.g., oncology, psychiatry); others by procedure (anesthesiology, radiology, surgery); others by age group (pediatrics, geriatrics). What does each specialty need to know about the subject of other specialties? Who really needs a general medical education? The extreme case is the psychiatrist. No wonder his post–medical school apprenticeship is so long; almost nothing in his medical school education is of any use to him in the practice of psychiatry. Only recently has a physiological component been added to his armamentarium, and even now the use of drugs is limited and in most cases a temporary treatment of symptoms, not a cure.

Not long ago, some of the procedural specialties in particular were not monopolized by M.D.s. Do they need an M.D. for reasons other than prestige and income? Of course what I am suggesting runs counter to every trend in education and professionalization. Specialists in pharmacology, genetics, virology, which are based on the structure of scientific investigation at this time, need not, perhaps should not, be M.D.s, but Ph.D.s. There is a need for generalists who can command teams of specialists as needed, not primary-care physicians whose internships are shorter than those of any specialty, who are typically regarded as a cut below the specialist. The generalist needed in a world of specialists is one whose training and experience more than match the specialist's, a specialist in diagnosis and in management of complex therapies, not necessarily a primary-care deliverer at all.

Half a century ago, the dedicated physician could master most of the useful medical knowledge of the time; a century ago, his stock of knowledge would remain little depreciated through his working life. Most of the useful instruments of his craft and the effective medications could be packed in a small black bag. That day is gone for good, and laments for the decline in the number and proportion of primary-care physicians are somewhat misplaced. The general practitioner is not competent to handle a wide range of problems up to the standards of modern medicine, nor will he or she have the equipment to do so. Much of the equipment now critical for diagnosis and treatment cannot be taken on house calls. Furthermore, no one can keep up with the progress of medicine across the board. Specialization is the inevitable consequence of the enormous expansion of knowledge and the growth of instrumentation and technique. It is also a consequence of scale: the fact that much medical care takes place in hospitals, where the division of labor increases productivity.

Until now, most of medicine has lacked a scientific base, in the sense of an understanding of the causes and conditions of health and disease and the functioning of therapeutic processes. Doctors are only now learning why aspirin, which has been in use most of this century, does what it does, and how; they are still discovering and examining hitherto unsuspected consequences of its regular use. We are now in the midst of an explosion of biochemistry, molecular biology, genetic experimentation and learning. Medicine is on its way toward acquiring a scientific base. The process is protracted, tortuous, complex; it quickly renders existing knowledge, or presumed knowledge, obsolete. New biochemical entities are identified or created at an alarming rate; new findings are challenged and techniques and therapies are modified or discarded. There is not time, in a general medical education, to get on top of the current state of knowledge in all medically relevant areas. There is not time in an active practice to keep up with new findings, tests, instruments, drugs, techniques, therapies.

To the extent that the role of the primary-care physician is to treat the more routine and minor conditions and refer others to specialists, it is not at all clear that he or she should have the same medical school training as other M.D.s. We need more primary-care physicians and fewer specialists, but it is not obvious that a large change in the ratio is called for. Nor is it clear that primary care should be monopolized by physicians. The division of labor between specialists, generalists, and paramedical personnel needs to be reconsidered and education and training revised accordingly.

Finally, we need a new kind of medical student and practitioner. The majority of medical students are driven by greed, not by service. The fact that most end up as specialists facilitates this transition from the older model of dedicated family physician. Given the extraordinarily high earnings for M.D.s that have prevailed for quite a few years, it is inevitable that medical schools should attract those driven mainly by greed. This has been true long enough that by now most doctors are among those thus motivated. They may all gainsay it, but it is unavoidable that this should be the case. The reluctance to specialize in primary care, which may be the most rewarding in terms of human relations, reflects the fact that primary-care physicians earn much less than most specialists, a fact well known to medical school students. If specialist medical earnings were to be cut by one-third, there would be a different breed of medical students, with a mentality much closer to the image of the family doctor than prevails today. And many more would choose to specialize in primary care.

Prices

Reduction in excess medical manpower will take decades. We cannot wait that long to do something about the excessive provision of services or about prices that are too high and rising too rapidly. Even if the market worked, it would take too long, and the verdict of the past is that competition in this industry raises prices. Competition is a problem, not a solution.

The relative value scales introduced by Medicare are a step in the right direction. They should be generalized to the entire health care supply covered by insurance. Perhaps relative prices should be biased in favor of primary-care physicians, as they have been in favor of specialists and procedures for many years. Relative value scales, which would narrow the income gap between general practitioners and most specialists, and lower the income of the latter, have two problems. First, if limited to Medicare, they reduce the number of specialists willing to accept Medicare patients. (They also reduce the quantity of overpriced services and procedures performed, and increase other services and procedures, which could be a good thing.) They can simply shift costs to other payers. The relative value scale must be applied across the board to all insurance coverage. But private insurance companies cannot do this severally, nor would they be allowed to collude to do it jointly. Second, a relative value scale is relative; overall incomes and expenditures remain too high. The entire scale must be recalibrated downward. It is a way of reducing the income differential between primary-care physicians and specialists, not by raising primary-care incomes, but by lowering specialist incomes. Few if any services or procedures or tests are underpaid in an absolute sense. But imposing a new scale with a lower base must be done gradually over a period of years. Equipment was acquired, hospitals were built, and doctors were educated and trained on the basis of prices that were and remain too high, and on the basis of relative prices skewed toward specialists, expensive equipment, and costly tests. We do not wish too many hospitals to close, or hospitals and specialists to engage in a desperate effort to increase services and procedures and cut quality to maintain income and cover costs, or too many young M.D.s unable to pay off the debts accumulated during their medical education and during the overworked and underpaid years as interns and residents. Income expectations will have to be lowered. Life is unfair, but it is in no one's interest to make it too unfair.

A schedule of relative prices, fees, charges should be established that will encourage primary care and discourage some specialties already in excess supply; eliminate insurance bias toward hospitalization in favor of outpatient treatment and home care; and encourage *cost-effective* prevention and early detection. (The last two objectives must also be promoted via insurance coverage.)

One reason for high prices is malpractice insurance. It is also a major justification for pressure to overtest, overtreat, and use the latest procedures and drugs. And it poisons the relation between doctor and customer. Efforts to limit expensive medical care to the very old, to the dying, to hopelessly deformed or handicapped neonatals, among others, where potential benefits are small and costs are large, rationing if you will, reserving available resources for those with much better prospects, will unquestionably lead to more malpractice claims. So will attempts to devise reasonable standards of medical treatment, say, in use of MRIs or fetal sonograms or caesarian sections. Inflated standards of practice initiated by opportunities for profit, and adopted for fear of malpractice, must be replaced. Since attorneys and their clients cannot be dissuaded from making outrageous demands, nor some juries from recommending preposterous compensation, limits must be set on the size of awards, as some states have already done, and on awards for unfavorable outcomes that are the result of neither negligence nor incompetence. Granted that the cases that make the news are atypical, very high insurance premiums are not, and their reduction is one requirement for lower prices, a requirement that should not affect M.D. incomes because the cost of malpractice insurance is fully passed on to the customer.

Insurance companies have tried to slow the rise in prices; HMOs have tried; Medicare has tried. HMOs and insurance companies have bargained with hospitals and other providers to lower prices for their clients. Medicare, with its captive clientele, imposed price (reimbursement) ceilings and expenditure ceilings (DRGs). The DRG system set a lid on expenditures but not on prices. Each has obtained concessions for its clientele, but the rise in prices shows no sign of a slowdown (but perhaps prices would have risen more in the absence of these determined efforts). The impact was on quantity, perhaps on quality. There are complaints that hospital patients are discharged too soon. Insurance companies, which have to compete with one another for clientele, have been slow to follow suit on DRG expenditure caps. The successes of some must have come at the expense of others because prices kept rising.

One factor in high and rising prices is the oversupply of hospital beds. Another is the oversupply in specialized equipment and facilities; too many MRIs, lithotriptors, cardiac surgery units. They are largely the consequence of competition. Underutilization of excess capacity raises costs and prices. Their use for unnecessary procedures may help keep prices down by spreading costs, but assures further growth in total expenditures.

There must be limits on prices. And there must be limits on the quantity of medical services. In fact we have had price "control" via Medicare and Medicaid for some time, but the total expenditures for these programs remain out of control for lack of sufficient quantity limitations. The more we reduce the number of new medical graduates and foreign-trained M.D.s, the more important it becomes to prevent prices from rising. As the surplus of M.D.s in many specialties is reduced, the opportunity to increase prices will improve, even though the workload and hence the income of the specialist should increase, given existing demand and prices. More urgently, as the supply of new medical graduates as cheap labor for hospitals is radically cut, hospitals will face higher labor costs and pressures to raise prices. Thus some leash on prices is needed to limit the side effects of reducing the surplus of M.D.s.

If the separate efforts of insurance companies and Medicare have not stopped the overall rise in prices and expenditures, a comprehensive approach is essential. Government price control is a scare phrase. Yet we accept the fact (or perhaps ignore the fact) that the utility rates we pay are set, not by firms, but by public utility commissions. God help us if the prices we had to pay for electricity and gas were set by the suppliers! The Federal Reserve Board sets interest rates that greatly influence all other interest rates, often over the objections of Congress, the executive branch, and business. I suggest that the public utility commission approach toward rate setting, with the independence of the Federal Reserve Board, is the way to go. It need not be a single national commission; it could be regional. There are substantial differences in nonmedical costs that should be reflected in prices. But local commissions run too high a risk of cooption. And they should set prices, as does Medicare through its relative value scale, not bargain over them; price levels are too high and relative prices are too distorted to be corrected by bargaining. A buyers' monopoly at the community level that negotiates insurance premiums or prepayment charges does not provide a set of relative prices that will both reduce costs substantially and alter incentives away from some specialties in oversupply. And how can it negotiate effectively with a supplier monopoly, as is common in smaller cities?

Earnings

Earnings in most cases should be reduced, but not by direct intervention. Limits on prices, changing relative prices to reduce the earnings differential between primary-care physicians and specialists, and limits on insurance coverage would bring down earnings. Reduced earnings where labor costs are a very large share of total costs, in medical schools and hospitals, would help reduce the costs of medical education and hospitalization (and counter the cost-increasing effects of a reduced supply of cheap interns and residents). Limits on quantity of medical services compensated by insurance become critically important as prices fall or fail to rise, for otherwise earnings are maintained by increasing the supply of services, as long as excess capacity continues to exist.

Nearly all goods and services are produced on the basis of workers earning wages and salaries, not individual fees. The fee-for-service system prevails in the absence of organized markets and for unstandardized, truly unique goods and services—new art products for instance. But these characteristics do not apply to the health care industry (the large industry of education does not operate on a fee-for-service basis). Education in many poor countries is partly fee for service for the wealthy: tutors. But in wealthy countries, where education is compulsory for all in fact as well as in word, fee for service has been replaced by salaried teachers. In countries, and in times, where most people never see a doctor, fee for service to the well-to-do prevails; but when medical care becomes a universal right, the fee-for-service market should become marginalized but not eliminated.

M.D.s on salary have no incentive to overtest, overtreat. They are under the surveillance of their fellow physicians. Freedom to set salaries at a reasonable level implies that fee for service must be a small part of medical care or must not be covered by insurance beyond average prices set in the salaried sector.

Elimination of surpluses in many specialties would increase the work-load of M.D.s in the fee-for-service market, which is much lower than in the HMO market, thus moderating declines in earnings as limits are set on prices and on their rates of increase (and increasing productivity). The expansion of HMOs and other group practices on a salaried basis would attract primary-care physicians disproportionately, reducing differences in pay between them and specialists, and increasing the surplus of specialists in the fee-for-service market. M.D.s should have an interest in reducing the inflow of new M.D.s into their specialties, even if hospitals and medical schools do not.

Coverage

One approach to quantity limitations is simply to specify which procedures are reimbursable and which are not. Again, Medicare and Medicaid do this, as do most private health insurance policies. Still, cost increases continue their runaway growth. The private firms must compete with one another and with the "Blues" and HMOs, and competition means more coverage, not less. To a limited extent, diagnoses and procedures can be altered to circumvent restrictions on reimbursement. But the main problem with negative lists is that they do not control quantity among tests and treatments that are approved. Control of quantity via micromanagement is out of the question; besides, it would impose a huge administrative cost on top of other costs.

A ceiling on total expenditures is not an adequate substitute, for it might mean a sharp decline in the quality of medical services: quantity would be sacrificed to maintain or increase already high prices and earnings, as we have observed in hospitals under DRGs. Quantity must be restricted, first by reducing the excess supply of physicians, hospital beds, and expensive equipment, which lead to excess supply of services and procedures. This will take decades, and we cannot wait.

We have to recognize that as long as health care seems to be free, there will be excessive demand; many people will not be satisfied. There is no solution to this problem. Restriction of coverage will reduce health insurance costs and reduce the quantity of uncovered services provided. It will not per se restrict the quantity of covered services; it provides no means of assuring that only those who need, who will benefit, from a service will receive it. Here we must rely on the professionalism of the M.D. As long as there is an economic incentive to offer unneeded services covered by insurance, some M.D.s will offer them. Medicare's DRG policy for hospitals, and HMOs, eliminate this incentive for their clientele.

Restriction of coverage refers, first, to conditions covered; second, to individuals eligible to receive coverage; and third, to technologies covered. As to conditions, first we rule out those for which treatment cannot be defined as health care. This of course implies a definition of health care, on which there will be much disagreement. One of the big issues is mental illness. This is not covered in many policies, and covered poorly in others. It is not just a matter of coverage, but of defining the disabilities covered. There is no dispute about schizophrenia and manic depression, but where do we draw the line on obsessive behavior, anxiety, irrational fears, and addictive behavior? Obesity, alcoholism, heroin addiction? What about nicotine addiction, recognized by the American Psychiatric Association? Another big issue is long-term care, also poorly provided for by nearly all policies. Where does health care end and custodial care take over? A third issue, just over the horizon, is the ability to test for dozens of serious genetic defects and in time to correct them. This will raise serious ethical as well as financial questions.

What technologies should be accepted for insurance coverage and taxpayer subsidy? Which should be available only at the patient's cost, if at all? Since the development of "halfway" technologies, which neither prevent nor cure, which are at best marginal improvements over existing technologies but typically much more costly, is a major cause of escalating medical costs, it is important to limit coverage to those that represent a significant gain in outcome or in risk or in cost. Next we exclude drugs and procedures that are not significant improvements over existing alternatives. Third, and most controversial, are procedures that incur intolerable costs. What is intolerable may depend on what the drug or procedures can accomplish, compared to alternatives, if any: prolong a life for a week, a month, a year? Prolong fully functional life or simply postpone death? Unfortunately, procedures cannot be simply classified according to these considerations. A respirator may allow damaged lungs to recover or may simply perpetuate life in a coma. We should also rule out procedures that involve high risks, except for patients who have little to lose, who would suffer permanent disability or die otherwise.

Ultimately, individual judgments on a case-by-case basis must be made on ruling out or accepting particular procedures. This raises another restriction on coverage: who should be eligible for high-cost or high-risk procedures or for procedures in short supply, such as organ transplants, which must be rationed, willing or not? Should alcoholics receive new livers, or heavy smokers new lungs? This question raises the emotional issue of behaviorally induced illness and its eligibility for coverage. How can we separate those who are faultless from those who brought serious illness on themselves? Besides, health care is for the sick, for whatever reason, like churches are for sinners, not just for saints. We can invest in behavior modification; illness is punishment enough.

The allocation of absolutely scarce goods, such as transplantable organs, is not a matter of cost, but of benefit. Age and physical condition should be considered. The economists' approach, the value of remaining expected life, based on lifetime earnings, has no popular or ethical support, but we should not lose sight of the fact that the losses, in terms of years of remaining life expectancy, are great for those who die young, often small for the elderly, who may not be said to have died prematurely.

Finally, what therapies (or practitioners) not falling under the aegis of the dominant allopathic medical establishment should be covered? Chiropractics, acupuncture, homeopathy?

Quality of Care

Most Americans believe that they are entitled to the best health care. But this is impossible; only a few can get the best.

Some physicians are better than others. Some hospitals are better than others. Given this ineluctable reality, only a small minority can get the best medical care. There are limits on ability to pay even to insurance companies, and limits on the willingness of government to pay, since ultimately it must tax its constituency to finance medical care. Thus the best medical care is available primarily for the rich.

Most people will never own a Mercedes Benz or drive a Rolls-Royce, nor is there any expectation that they should. Yet in medical care many feel that we are all entitled to Rolls-Royces. "Medicine concerns the inalienable right of each individual to enjoy the healthiest, most disease-free body that state-of-the-art knowledge allows. In its commitment to that right, the practice of medicine has stood apart from the values of the marketplace."[4] But one of the implications of limited income is a limited ability to pay, and also a limited willingness to transfer income via taxation to others so that they may pay. The same writer adds, many pages later, that "most observers agree that the country can no longer afford the kind of medical care to which it has become accustomed." But habits are hard to break.

Health, and therefore health care, is not the only "need" we consider important. In 1938 we passed the Fair Labor Standards Act establishing a minimum wage of 25 cents an hour, which has since been raised to $4.25. We did not specify that everyone should have even excellent wages. For those without sufficient income, we give food stamps. They can provide an adequate healthy diet but not champagne and caviar, not gourmet meals. We have to pay for these without help from the government or anyone else. We provide housing subsidies, but not for mansions, or even for four bedrooms, three baths, and a swimming pool in the backyard. These we can own only if we can afford them. In education, we do not offer most schoolchildren excellent schools, the best education. That they must pay for, or earn entry through scholarly achievement. Why in the world should health care be different? "A guaranteed level of healthcare is only sensible financially, and only feasible politically, if there are firm limits to the individual demands that can be made for medical cures."[5] Those who want more, or better, should pay.

Because of the individualized nature of health care delivery, the long gaps in personal experience for most individuals, and the lack of or ignorance of performance standards with wide applicability, awareness of the problem of quality was a long time coming, and, for the same reasons, concern about quality is likely to remain an irritant in patient–health care industry relations long after cause for concern has disappeared. Unfortunately, competitive pressure and comparison shopping, which shocked the lethargic auto industry into a desperate struggle for survival in the face of Japanese competition, works later and more slowly in an industry such as health care. The discipline imposed by foreign competition in the case of autos is being enforced by a growing surplus of hospitals and M.D.s in the years ahead. Hospitals and M.D.s will have to compete vigorously for patients. Many have overcome their reluctance to advertise, their strange view that the normal process of bringing information to the attention of customers in other industries was "unethical" for doctors and hospitals. The more information that can be provided to prospective customers on the quality of practitioners and institutions, the more efficient can this competition become in raising the quality of medical care.

Insurance

The fact that many millions do not have access to group rates for health insurance means that millions choose not to purchase health insurance because their income is adequate, but they are healthy, mostly young; their needs are few; millions pay rates close to twice those they would pay had they access to group or community rates. Providing such rates to all would reduce total expenditures for health insurance for those who pay individual rates and would reduce the number not covered, as many buy policies at the reduced rates. Some of those already covered by individual policies would opt for higher-benefit policies than they now hold. On the other hand, tax subsidies for policies through employers may lead to excessive insurance and misinform workers about the price they are paying. The employees, not the employers, pay.

How to break the link between insurance and escalating costs of medical care? A single payer would greatly reduce administrative costs, but this is a once-and-for-all saving. Ours is the most expensive bureaucracy in the world by a wide margin, adding some 20 percent to health care costs. A single payer could mean standardization of prices, could mean their reduction, and would permit standardization of coverage. It could offer more than one option in terms of co-payments, in terms of deductibles, and for that matter, in terms of coverage. It would mean an end to the vicious circle of competitive escalation of prices and quantities between insurance companies. Price schedules could be designed to encourage correcting regional imbalances.

Standardized forms would reduce administrative costs somewhat even with 1,500 payers. Standard reimbursement across the industry would make comparisons easier; it can be accomplished only through the intervention of government. Insurers could still compete in coverage, deductibles, co-payments. Standard coverage would further standardize forms, save a little on administrative costs, and limit competition to co-payments and deductibles. These are the elements of competition most comprehensible to the general public. A fee-for-service medical sector would survive, but it is important that it not be allowed to drive up salaries in the prepayment sector (HMOs) or compel the prepayment sector to compete in expensive technology of questionable advantage over older and cheaper alternatives.

Research and Development

Price levels and relative prices alone may not guarantee desired results. Strict control over procedures to be covered, and individual eligibility for covered procedures, must be monitored, or the effects of lower prices on costs will surely be circumvented by higher quantities. The most important aspect of quantity control is the evaluation of new technologies. Introduction of "halfway" technologies should be minimized; and use and reimbursement for any new technology should be limited to those likely to benefit significantly. Risk-reward, or cost-benefit guidelines are needed. Standards need to be developed for the use of and reimbursement for screening and testing in general, to avoid indiscriminate mass screening and testing, especially for genetic propensities for disease.

Research and development need not be cut back, might perhaps be expanded but redirected from halfway technologies, from politically driven applied research projects unlikely to produce worthwhile results toward the basic research needed before applied research and development can pay off; toward cost-reducing process innovations and away from cost-increasing product innovations. Not all halfway technologies need be denied coverage; some of them represent big improvements in outcome, or large reductions in medical or economic costs. Nor should we forget that some halfway technologies represent a significant advance toward successful prevention or treatment.

Restriction of coverage for halfway technologies implies a change in FDA priorities in approval of new drugs, new instruments and materials. Since 1962, the FDA has been obsessed with safety, which can never be assured before years of actual experience, even though the United States has the strictest requirements in the world. They should be relaxed, and procedures for systematic collection of postintroduction data should be established. Mistakes will be made, whatever the process. Reducing excessive and overly long testing requirements for approval may require some change in personnel, with responsibility for decisions shifted to individuals whose reputations and careers do not hang in the balance—consultants perhaps, rather than career civil servants. Efficacy should not be a sufficient criterion for approval. A new drug or material or instrument must be significantly superior to existing alternatives in outcome or in safety or cost.

If it is true that the remaining health problems are genetic, environmental, or lifestyle in origin, then the health research agenda for the future is quite different from that of the past when microorganisms were the dominant cause of disease. The remaining unknown or unsolved problems of health call for research. This has always been true, but now appears to be one of the times when we are on a near plateau, higher of course than the plateaus of prevention and treatment attained in the past. Most of the gains from prevention and from treatment have already been achieved, within the limits of existing knowledge. The research called for is new in emphasis: much more statistical analysis of vast bodies of data to identify key factors from among an enormous variety of circumstances. It will be done by different kinds of researchers. The "cures" that have been and will be forthcoming are likewise quite different from those originating in drug companies and medical schools, NIH and universities. For example, a major "cure" for sulfate air pollution is stack scrubbers; for other pollutants, catalytic converters or a change in fuel composition; also, food additives to avoid various mineral and vitamin deficiencies. Among the "cures" for ailments of genetic origin or predisposition is genetic counseling. Such "cures" depend both on research findings and on information and education of the public and legislatures in the case of environmental protection measures, of parents and would-be parents in the case of genetic counseling. Finally, the matter of lifestyle: since it is not the only factor correlated with health and disease, nor entirely deterministic, it is extraordinarily difficult to establish the facts and relations, to prescribe, to convince, and this is a job mainly carried out by individuals and institutions not normally regarded as part of the health and medical industry. Once the facts and relations are established, there remains the enormous job of information and the persuasion of 260 million people.

In the future, research and information should focus much more on public health measures as exemplified by EPA, which confronts nonmicrobiotic or parasitic sources of disease, and particularly on private health measures carried out by individuals and not by the medical care establishment. Information is the task of school systems, the various media, the press in particular.

What about the remaining major medical burdens of illness and poor health? Heart and arteriosclerotic disease, cancer, arthritis, allergies, Alzheimer's, and osteoporosis in most cases do not fit the germ model of disease. Most of the remaining burden of disease is of genetic origin or predisposition, or environmental, or behavioral in origin. For most of the resulting ailments there is no magic bullet, and for some there may never be. Drugs or surgery may to some extent counteract or correct for many long-standing behavioral abuses, or pollutant exposures, but there is no prospect that in the future we will be able to behave in any way we choose with impunity, whether collectively in polluting the environment or individually in neglecting simple rules of good health.

The enormous achievements in prevention and the great strides in treatment are mostly the result of scientific research and development. The achievements of research are permanent, whereas most prevention and treatment requires continuing resources, sustained effort. But research is not a one-way process from lab to M.D. If enough effort is devoted to pooling the experience of many physicians, valid conclusions are obtainable. Most physicians do not participate in such an effort to assess outcomes. There are no incentives to do so, nor any requirements. The computers and software that permit easy and prompt dissemination of new medical knowledge are also useful in collecting and analyzing the data on which it is based.

Competition

Competition does not work in the market for medical care, and I do not think it can be made to work. If it did, competition between hospitals in large metropolitan areas with many empty beds would result in lower prices. If there were effective competition, earnings and fees in specialties in excess supply would fall relative to those of primary-care physicians. The opposite has happened. The surplus of specialists and the shortage of generalists has worsened, but the difference in earnings has widened. Relative prices differ widely, often by a multiple, from relative value indices, which reflect costs, including time, training, and difficulty. That means monopoly power and monopoly profits. How does an increasing surplus lead to rising incomes? Specialization, in conjunction with closed hospital staff privileges and the referral system from primary-care physicians, effectively creates considerable monopoly power; the specialist has considerable latitude in raising prices. To the extent that costs are covered by insurance, the customer does not care

With third-party payments and fee for service, competition for customers is not, cannot be, in price. It must be in quantity, quality, or both; any of which results in cost increases. Only with ceilings on total reimbursement can competition be in price. And experience shows that reimbursement caps result in reduced quantity of services: shorter hospital stays, rather than lower prices. Such ceilings are more effective for hospitals than for individual M.D.s.[6] In hospitals there are internal pressures from medical staff to obtain the latest equipment, perform new procedures, prescribe the latest drugs. The individual physician does not see any conflict between his or her income and the purchase of the latest and best, even though the conflict is obvious to management. There is external pressure: subscribers and even employers also want the latest and the best. Under these conditions, the more competition, the higher the costs and prices. Even HMOs, as long as they face competition from fee-for-service medical care, have limited ability to compete on reimbursement of medical personnel; the salaries they must pay to attract and hold personnel are set in the fee-for-service market; to some extent so are the quantity and quality of services they must render.

Competition fails because, with insurance coverage, the consumer is insensitive to cost; but also because of consumer ignorance. The consumer cannot judge the need nor the quality of care; he or she does not know most medical costs in advance, other than routine office visits; which or how many tests will be ordered by the physician, or what procedures will be recommended. Under these circumstances, consumer demand is not independent but is determined by the supplier, the M.D. If there is an oversupply of providers and facilities, their influence will be reflected in additional demand from customers.

A growing share of Americans with health care coverage are enrolled in groups. The large employer providing health insurance for employees does shop around, does seek to keep costs down, contracting with groups that have an incentive to keep costs below the contract price. But HMO costs rise just as fast as those of the fee-for-service market.

Underlying the ineffectiveness, or counterproductivity, of competitive pressure is the technological imperative on the side of the professional and the demand for more and better on the part of the customer, who is not prepared to settle for what he or she can afford, or for second best, even though that is what happens in consumption behavior everywhere else. As long as health care is free, too much will be demanded.

Somehow the link between third-party payments and other elements of cost increase must be severed. It can be accomplished only by reorganizing the delivery of medical care to provide an incentive to the provider to avoid excessive testing and treatment, to limit excessive acquisition of the latest equipment and prescription of the latest drugs, removing the incentive for research and development of new drugs and equipment that represent little or no improvement over existing alternatives. Competition will not accomplish this; on the contrary, it will exacerbate the problem. An HMO provides these incentives, unless it faces competition from independent providers or other HMOs, which compel it to engage in cost-increasing competition and to pay higher salaries. The health care market simply is not well enough informed, and never can be, as long as the customer can make decisions. Most employers are not much better informed and lack the incentives to serve as agents for their employees.

It may be more realistic to treat the medical care industry as a public utility, as a natural monopoly, rather than as a potentially perfectly competitive industry. The monopoly arises not from the causes found in public utilities, although in smaller cities the economies-of-scale argument is not absent, but from the inability of the customer to make informed choices for two reasons: lack of ability to make judgments, and bias toward more and more expensive care arising from third-party payments. Such bias is unavoidable and is reducible only by forcing the customer to pay a large share of the costs, that is, by limiting third-party payments. We do not want to do this, in part because of its adverse impact on low-income people.

The public utility approach toward regulating health care is not new. We already do this to some extent, through the Food and Drug Administration. The purpose is not to avoid excessive prices charged by a natural monopolist; in fact, excessive prices are often charged. The purpose is to protect the public from dangers to health and life from which the public is incapable of protecting itself, and in fact even individual M.D.s are incapable of protecting all their customers. The issue is information about the benefits of a drug and the risks of using it. The FDA is protecting the public from pharmaceutical companies that might sell drugs offering no benefit and drugs the risks of which are unknown or excessive in view of the benefits; not from excessive profits, but excessive risks of harmful side effects; not from monopoly of production, although this may exist, but monopoly of information, or lack of information. The FDA does not set rates or rates of return, but decides which drugs may be sold and for which uses they may be prescribed. (Once approval is granted for the sale of a drug, it is nearly impossible to see that it is used only for the allowed uses.) Even after approval, the FDA regulates information that must be made available to all users about the proper uses of the drug, its counterindications, its possible side effects.

Competition cannot cope with quantity: how much of approved procedures at approved prices will be conducted? This kind of micromanagement has to be left to health care providers, thus the need to favor organizations of health care that have incentives to limit provision to clearly beneficial services.

A fee-for-service medical sector would survive, but it is important that it not be allowed to drive up salaries in the prepayment sector or preclude them from declining in real terms as appropriate; that it not compel the prepayment sector to compete in expensive technology or drugs of questionable advantage over older and cheaper alternatives, or for inappropriate uses.

A buyers' monopoly at the community level negotiates insurance premiums or prepayment charges. It does not provide a set of relative prices that will both reduce costs substantially and alter incentives toward primary care and away from specialties in oversupply.

Productivity

What is the productivity of the health care industry, and how will the suggestions above for its reform affect productivity? A complete measure of productivity in the medical industry requires information on outcomes; costs of medical care; externalities via contribution of health care to labor-force participation, productivity, hence economic output and economic growth. We propose to consider only the first two.

Infant mortality and life expectancy are two crude measures of productivity. But whose productivity? Much of the gains must be allocated to public health. How much is a medical contribution? We have specific measures, such as hospital bed days, but they are pure input measures. We need output measures: how do heart attack victims or cancer victims fare as a result of a variety of treatments? Even if we had output measures, they say nothing about the rate of heart attacks or the rate of various kinds of cancers. Health care should also be concerned with the incidence of cancers, the rate of heart attacks, not just their treatment. Health care that reduces the incidence of illness is as pertinent a component of productivity as health care that promotes recovery. We know a lot more about treatment than about the determinants of the incidence of many illnesses and ways of reducing the incidence, hence the stress on specific output measures. The morbidity rate determinants are diverse. Some are medical strategies proper: drugs for high blood pressure, diabetes, allergies, which may constitute treatment but also prevention. Others are public health measures: chlorination and fluoridation of water supplies, air-pollution controls, vaccination, food safety controls, antismoking regulations. Yet others are not normally placed under the rubric of public health, although that is where they belong, for example, workplace safety. Then there is private health care: no smoking, safe driving, sound lifestyle. These things can reduce the productivity of the health care industry.

The nonmedical component of health care costs is also growing. The main cost is not in government budgets but in increased cost of production of a wide range of goods and services. The measure of such widely distributed increased costs is in a slower increase in productivity (in some cases a decline) and a slower growth of GNP, but measuring it is next to impossible. Estimation of the benefits, such as those of reduced air pollution, is also very difficult and very rough; they are statistical lives saved, illness reduced, rather than specific individuals benefiting from treatment. It is safe to say that much of the effort of EPA and OSHA imposes unnecessarily large costs on the community and yields minimal benefits; risks are grossly exaggerated, costs underestimated. Their contribution to health is small, and their negative contribution to the economy is substantial; their productivity is negative.

But even in regard to medical costs, one can ask, had the resources not been expended in health care, how would they have been used, and what would have been the resulting increase in productivity and GNP? Comparing productivity of diverse procedures and programs that save lives is relatively easy. How much does it cost to save one life? The range of costs is enormous, from a few hundred dollars to many millions. Which should be funded? How much is a life worth? But most of the benefits of health care, and environmental improvement, are not measured in reduced mortality but reduced morbidity. Here rank ordering is more complex, since there are many gradations of morbidity, none easily measured, only one of mortality. Crude comparisons in terms of days lost from work or bed days can be made. But there is strong resistance to "rationing" health care on the basis of who will be likely to benefit most.

The differences in availability of health care resources (M.D.s, hospital beds) between states are enormous, but the differences in infant mortality and in longevity are minimal, suggesting that differences in medical resources, within the range experienced in the United States, make little difference, that the productivity of additional medical resources is extremely low. Should more resources be devoted to prevention? Traditional prevention would not contribute much more than it already does to reducing mortality and morbidity were it to receive large additional funds. What about the new public health of EPA and related agencies? It may be decades before we can be reasonably assured of the magnitude of their contribution, or of the benefits of additional investments in these areas, but the evidence to date is not encouraging. Efforts to inform the public and motivate it to take preventive lifestyle measures are hard to evaluate.

Much of our medical resources are invested in treatments for which there is no scientific justification, despite statements by medical and scientific lobbies to the contrary. There is no evidence that they are beneficial or that the medical benefits outweigh the medical risks (never mind the ratio of economic costs to economic benefits). We can justify this statement by examining clinical studies comparing differences in outcomes of treated and untreated control groups; by comparing outcomes in the United States, where patients are treated, with outcomes in other countries, where similar patients are not treated.

One example of irrational allocation of resources to health is the failure to vaccinate millions of pre-school-age children. A second is the bias toward hospitalization because outpatient treatment may not be reimbursed by insurance companies. A third is recourse to a physician when a nurse or a counselor would be adequate, if not better, for the same reason. A fourth is medical education, which requires the same long training for all students, even though those choosing some specialties will find little use for most of their medical school education. The small proportion of graduates in primary-care specialties is another example of misallocation. There are too many caesarean sections, too much medication for marginally elevated serum cholesterol and for marginally elevated blood pressure, far too many coronary bypasses—in fact too much surgery in general—too much life-extension treatment for very elderly people and others with no prospect of recovering to useful lives, and not enough prenatal care. How do we know? Not just by comparing rates in the United States with rates in other advanced nations, but by examining the need, the net benefits, including the risks.

Treatment for what? Contagious and infectious diseases not eliminated or greatly reduced by preventive measures can be classified into those readily treatable by available antibiotics, and those, mainly viral diseases, that cannot be so treated. A growing share of the workload of hospitals, by now the major share, has little to do with infections by microorganisms: cancer, stroke, heart and circulatory system disease, mental illness, allergies, metabolic problems. For some of these conditions we lack effective treatments. Some are not fully reversible, and the optimal strategy now and for the foreseeable future appears to be prevention. But our knowledge about prevention is inadequate.

In research, too much is spent to develop drugs that are at best marginally different from existing drugs, and then too much is spent on advertising to gain market share in crowded therapeutic markets. There is excessive duplication of research and development by pharmaceutical firms. Federal funds are subject to political pressures, rather than therapeutic priorities. What is not realized when there are demands for yet more spending is that there is a limited number of highly qualified researchers, and this number cannot be expanded in the short run no matter how much is spent, so the effect is diversion.

The average M.D. spends a lot less time as chauffeur, clerk, and low-level technician and much more as a practicing physician. Thus M.D. productivity must have gained considerably with urbanization, improved transportation and communication, and the demise of house calls, except by telephone. The average M.D. now has the assistance of many times more health workers than before, as well as expensive equipment and facilities. One has to include their cost in estimating productivity. The increasing surplus in the past twenty years implies a decline in productivity. Many specialists are underworked and supply too many unnecessary services and procedures. A reduction in surplus should increase productivity both by increasing their workload and by reducing that part of their current workload that yields minimal if any benefit, whose product is zero or close to it.

The large increase in hospital personnel per occupied bed over the past two decades suggests a decline in productivity also, unless it can be shown that there was enough improvement in outcomes to justify the additional cost. A reduction in the number of available hospital beds, in the number of hospital personnel, and in the number of costly facilities and equipment will reduce costs and improve productivity.[7]

One cannot speak of the productivity of any health care sector without considering the contribution of other sectors. Good public health, clean environment, and sound health habits reduce the productivity of medical care by eliminating the need for some of the most productive interventions. Conversely, good diagnosis and treatment minimize the harm done by a polluted environment or poor health habits and therefore the benefit from environmental policies or behavioral modification. Survival of much of the population into their seventies and eighties means that medical care shifts attention toward chronic conditions that cannot be cured and that successful interventions extend life and health a few years, not a few decades. Thus medical productivity is declining. The same is true of other sectors of health care. Once people have been persuaded to give up smoking, there is nothing else they can do that will improve their health and life expectancy nearly as much. Once the belching smokestacks and exhaust pipes are cleaned up, lead removed from paint and fuels, the population vaccinated against highly infectious and dangerous diseases, and the water supply chlorinated, what is there left for an encore that is not anticlimactic? Nothing of course is more creative than a lobby without a cause; new hazards, new illnesses will be invented if not discovered. Nevertheless, health care is facing diminishing returns, and it is hard to believe that any research breakthroughs can restore productivity to the levels reached during the early decades of the antibiotic revolution. At what point is the productivity of additional investment in medical care or environmental safety or changes in lifestyle so low that it is not worth the additional cost?

Diminishing returns from further investments in treatment and prevention suggest diminishing returns from additional research and development as well, until there are major breakthroughs in treating remaining major sources of morbidity and mortality. Mortality is already so low until age sixty, with the exception of AIDS, that remaining gains are bound to be limited until such time as means are found to extend the useful life span, as distinguished from treating the conditions and illnesses of the aged. No one knows when such breakthroughs temporarily reversing the inexorable trend of diminishing returns will occur, nor how much in research they will cost. Until then, increasing expenditures for medical care cannot be justified in terms of health benefits and risks, never mind the economic costs of health gains. The costs are not just money, they are other desiderata foregone.

* * *

There is no single, simple solution. What is needed if the share of GNP devoted to health care is to fall to more reasonable levels, and be kept there, is a combination of a large reduction in the number of medical personnel and facilities; a list of services for which there is no insurance coverage, plus price ceilings on services that are covered; a shift of incentives away from overprovision of services toward limiting them to instances of medical need and worth; and, perhaps, an overall spending ceiling, to limit the quantity of covered services provided. The latter spending ceiling requires reorganization of the delivery of medical care. It can be applied to HMOs and similar systems of prepaid delivery of health care that have an incentive to restrain spending. It can be imposed on hospitals, by generalizing Medicare's DRG system, with payment depending on the diagnostic classification. It is not workable in fee-for-service health care delivery.

How can all of this come about? There must be a profound change in attitudes toward individual rights. No individual has the right to empty another's pocket; but that is precisely what is widely believed, and often practiced: theft by another name. Rights to health care are social, not individual, and must be defined by a process of consensus. This is what we do in signing an insurance contract of any kind, or joining an HMO; the signer has limited rights: to specific services, under specific conditions, to limited amounts. The citizen pays taxes not of his choice, receives benefits also not as he chooses, but as the body politic specifies. The rights of any individual are limited by the rights of others. Health care is no exception.

Notes

1. Richard Lamm, "What It Will Take to Really Control Health Care Costs," *Medical Economics*, July 20, 1992, 81–89.

2. Victoria McEvoy, "Medical School Still Doesn't Prepare Us to Be Doctors," *Medical Economics* 70, no. 10 (May 24, 1993).

3. Daniel Greenberg, "Medical Walter Mittys," *Washington Post*, June 5, 1979, A17.

4. Stanley Wohl, *The Medical Industrial Complex* (New York: Harmony Books, 1984), 6.

5. Daniel Callahan, *What Kind of Life: The Limits of Medical Progress* (New York: Simon and Schuster, 1990), 28; see also 32.

6. Gregory Pope, "Physician Inputs, Outputs and Productivity, 1976–1986," *Inquiry* 27 (Summer 1990): 151–60.

7. Jerry Crowell and Gregory Pope, "Trends in Hospital Labor and Total Factor Productivity," *Health Care Financing Review* (Summer 1989): 39; John Ashby and Stuart Altman, "The Trend in Hospital Output and Labor Productivity," *Journal of the American Medical Association* 29 (Spring 1992): 80–91.

Index

About the Author

Charles T. Stewart, Jr., is Professor of Economics Emeritus at George Washington University, where he taught for many years. He has also been a research economist at the U.S. Chamber of Commerce. Professor Stewart specializes in the economics of human resources: technological change, health, and education. Among his many books are *Technology Transfer and Human Factors* (1987), which won the Ohira Memorial Prize; *From Basic Economics to Supply Side Economics* (1983) and *Economics for the Voter* (1981), both written with Melvin Greenhut; and *Air Pollution, Human Health, and Public Policy* (1979).